CLOCK DRAWING

CLOCK DRAWING

A Neuropsychological Analysis

Morris Freedman, M.D., F.R.C.P. (C)
Larry Leach, Ph.D.
Edith Kaplan, Ph.D.
Gordon Winocur, Ph.D.
Kenneth I. Shulman, M.D., F.R.C.P. (C)
Dean C. Delis, Ph.D

New York   Oxford
OXFORD UNIVERSITY PRESS
1994

Oxford University Press

Oxford   New York   Toronto
Delhi   Bombay   Calcutta   Madras   Karachi
Kuala Lumpur   Singapore   Hong Kong   Tokyo
Nairobi   Dar es Salaam   Cape Town
Melbourne   Auckland   Madrid

and associated companies in
Berlin   Ibadan

Library of Congress Cataloging-in-Publication Data
Clock drawing : a neuropsychological analysis /
Morris Freedman . . . [et al.].
p.   cm. Includes bibliographical references and index.
ISBN 0-19-505906-9
1. Neuropsychological tests.   2. Brain damage–Diagnosis.
3. Dementia–Diagnosis.   4. Cognition disorders–Diagnosis.
5. Alzheimer's disease–Diagnosis.   I. Freedman, Morris, 1949–
[DNLM: 1. Neuropsychological Tests.
2. Brain Diseases–diagnosis.   3. Cognition Disorders–diagnosis.
WM 145 C643 1994] RC386.6.N48C55   1994
616.8'0475–dc20
DNLM/DLC for Library of Congress   93-13481

9 8 7 6 5 4 3 2 1

Printed in the United States of America
on acid-free paper

Preface

The motivation to write this book arose from the need to establish normative data for the assessment of clock drawing in both elderly and young adults. In addition, we wanted to provide a practical guide to help clinicians and researchers analyze the broad variety of abnormal clocks drawn by patients with dementia and focal brain lesions, as well as to develop an easy-to-administer scoring system for quantitative assessment of clock drawing. To accomplish our goals, we conducted a normative study of clock drawing in a large sample of normal subjects ranging in age from 20 to 90 years. The findings are described in Chapter 2, along with data about the construct validity, specificity, and sensitivity of the clock-drawing task. Our relatively simple quantitative scoring system for the assessment of clock drawing is also presented.

In Chapter 1 we discuss the concept of clock drawing as a neuropsychological test instrument and highlight the need to select the most sensitive time setting for bringing out deficits. We emphasize the clinical importance of asking patients to draw clocks both to command and to copy, as well as the relevance of using different clock conditions. We also stress the value of using a process-oriented approach for obtaining a fine clinical analysis, although we recognize that a quantitative scoring system is appropriate as an initial screen.

Chapter 3 focuses on the clocks drawn by patients with dementia due to disorders such as Alzheimer's and Parkinson's disease. A section on the use of clock drawing for longitudinal follow-up of dementia has also been included. In addition, we describe clock-drawing ability in other disorders of cognitive function including metabolic encephalopathy, traumatic brain injury, and disconnection syndromes.

Chapter 4 describes clock-drawing ability in cognitively intact elderly individuals who are living in a supportive environment for reasons other than intellectual impairment. This chapter not only compares the clocks of the elderly in a seniors' residence to those of individuals living in the community but also provides insights into the changes in clock drawing that may represent the earliest markers of cognitive decline in the elderly.

The final chapter describes clock drawing after focal brain lesions and illustrates the differences in the errors produced by patients with left versus right hemisphere lesions and those with anterior versus posterior lesions. This chapter also highlights the concept that clock drawing is not only a sensitive measure of cognitive dysfunction due to lesions in different sites but also that the profile of deficits on this task may reflect the different types of damage that may result in brain disease.

Our aim is to provide clinicians and researchers with a better understanding of clock drawing in patients with cognitive dysfunction and to stimulate new ideas for the innovative use of clock drawing as a neuropsychological test instrument.

Toronto   M. F.
May 1993   L. L.
                                                                                                          E. K.
                                                                                                          G. W.
                                                                                                       K. I. S.
                                                                                                       D.C.D.

Acknowledgments

We gratefully acknowledge Stephanie Bernstein Covall, Reesa Hotz-Sud and Catherine Lanneval for their commitment, persistence, and many hours of tireless work spent testing subjects, analyzing data and assisting with preparation of the manuscript. In addition, we also greatly appreciate the assistance provided by Lee Ferreira-Hutzol, Karen Saeger and Tania Sherri-Cattle with data analysis, preparation of figures, and other help. We owe special thanks to Vicki Giardino whose dedication and efforts in preparing the manuscript were without equal.

The cooperation of our many colleagues who referred patients for testing is gratefully acknowledged.

We would also like to express our appreciation to Jeffrey House, Oxford University Press, for his advice and helpful suggestions for the preparation of the manuscript.

The research reported in this manuscript was supported in part by research grants from the Medical Research Council of Canada (Drs. Freedman and Winocur), the Ontario Mental Health Foundation (Dr. Freedman), and the Canadian Federal Government's Networks of Centers of Excellence Program (Drs. Freedman and Winocur), as well as Career Scientist Award from the Ministry of Health of Ontario to Dr. Freedman.

Contents

CLOCK DRAWING

1. Introduction

For decades, clock-drawing tasks have been used to assess the mental status of patients with various neurologic or psychiatric disorders (Critchley, 1953; Luria, 1980; Mayer-Gross, 1935; Schuell, 1965; Van der Horst, 1934; Warrington, James, & Kinsborne, 1966). Clock drawing continues to enjoy widespread use in clinical practice (Albert & Kaplan, 1980; Benton, 1985a; Eddy & Sriram, 1977; Goodglass & Kaplan, 1979, 1983; Heilman & Valenstein, 1985; Kaplan, 1988, 1990; Lezak, 1983; Weintraub & Mesulam, 1985; Strub & Black, 1985) and has experienced a recent resurgence in interest (Henderson, Mack, & Williams, 1989; Libon, Swensen, Barnoski, & Sands, 1993; Rouleau, Salmon, Butters, Kennedy, & McGuire, 1992; Sunderland, Hill, Mellow, Lawlor, Gundersheimer, Newhouse, & Grafman, 1989; Tuokko, Hadjistavropoulos, Miller, & Beattie, 1992; Wolf-Klein, Silverstone, Levy, & Brod, 1989).

Many authors use clock drawing as a test of visuoconstructive abilities (e.g., Albert & Kaplan, 1980; Andrews, Brocklehurst, Richards, & Laycock, 1980; Battersby, Bender, Pollack, & Kahn, 1956; Lezak, 1983; Weintraub & Mesulam, 1985; Spreen & Strauss, 1991). Other investigators have placed emphasis on clock reading or setting as a means of evaluating symbolic representation (e.g., Head, 1926; Mayer-Gross, 1935; McFie & Zangwill, 1960; Van der Horst, 1934), while others stress the use of clock drawing as a means of assessing executive or praxic functions (e.g., Luria, 1980; Mayer-Gross, 1935). These various functions that clock drawing as a visuospatial task is presumed to tap and the various brain regions thought to subserve these functions derive from ideas that were generated over the past century (for a review of this period see Benton, 1985a).

Historically, visuospatial perception involving visual recognition and memory was associated with the posterior region of the right hemisphere of the brain (Jackson, 1874). At the turn of the century, Liepmann proposed a disconnection syndrome (lateralized to the left hemisphere) to account for the apraxias (see Geschwind, 1975). At about that time, a number of German neurologists proposed an apraxia, or disconnection syndrome, as the mechanism to account for some specific visuospatial disorders.

For example, Kleist (1912) attributed impaired constructional spatial ability involved in drawing to "constructional apraxia" localized to the parieto-occipital region of the left or dominant hemisphere. Poppelreuter (1917) proposed the term "visual apraxia" (localized to either or both occipital lobes) to account for visuomotor deficits that included such visuoconstructional impairments as copying designs. In the strict sense, the term *apraxia* implies a disorder of skilled movement due to a disconnection between brain regions mediating perception and primary motor function. Moreover, this disconnection occurs in a setting where primary perceptual and motor functions are intact. Nevertheless, the frequent findings of perceptual deficits in association with "constructional problems" did not discourage the use of Kleist's term "constructional apraxia." (It would be more correct to substitute "impairment" for apraxia.) What did come under fire, however, was Kleist's attribution of dysfunction lateralized to the left hemisphere of the brain. Evidence was mounting to account for visuospatial and visuoconstructive problems in association with lesions lateralized to the right cerebral hemisphere. Though lesions of the right hemisphere resulted in more severe impairments, constructional problems could also occur with lesions lateralized to the left hemisphere. The diplomatic speculation was that there were two distinctive types of constructional impairment. One was due to dysfunction in the left hemisphere producing a motor execution constructional disability, whereas the other was due to a disordered right hemisphere causing deficits in visuospatial perceptual processing. Piercy and Smyth (1962) could not confirm such speculation. Their study concluded that there was bilateral but unequal visuospatial representation in the two hemispheres.

Within the last decades, however, results from split-brain research and focal lesion studies have clarified the distinctive role played by the two cerebral hemispheres—as well as specific regions within each hemisphere—in visuospatial information processing (Kaplan, 1988). The drawing of a clock is a task that permits an appreciation of the various ways visuospatial functions may be compromised.

Component Functions

Ostensibly, drawing a clock is a simple task. Nonetheless, it is a task that requires contributions from diverse cerebral regions. In the presence of brain injury or disease, some relevant functions are often compromised. The patient's final production often represents an interaction between his or her selective deficits and the struggle to compensate using those functions that are spared. Thus, the nature of a patient's clock-drawing impairment can vary greatly depending on the type and location of the pathology.

When given the verbal command to "draw a clock," an individual must possess adequate auditory language skills to comprehend the instructions. There must also be a representation of the visuospatial features of a clock as well as a mechanism for retrieving this knowledge. In addition, visuoperceptual and visuomotor processes are needed to translate the mental representation into a motor program for drawing. Visual perception guides the spatial layout of the component features of a clock, and hemi-attentional processes ensure that the features are represented accurately in both sides of space. Visual perception also monitors the motor output, and corrections are made via control processes of executive functions. The linguistic system is also called upon at output to provide the graphomotor representation of the clock numbers. It is this aspect that gives drawing a clock the advantage over drawing a daisy or a house.

In clock drawing, some cognitive processes must operate in parallel—i.e., the patient must write the numbers while simultaneously maintaining their correct spatial layout with regard to all the numbers and the relation of the numbers to the contour of the clock. Executive functions of planning, organization, and simultaneous processing are thus required to coordinate the multiple steps. If the task includes instructions for a specific time setting, then memory skills are needed to store and later retrieve the time setting after the clock face and numbers have been drawn. These diverse component skills are differentially organized in cortical and subcortical, anterior and posterior, and left and right cerebral hemispheres. Each component can be selectively impaired, resulting in a qualitatively distinct drawing. It is this sampling of multiple neurocognitive functions that makes the clock-drawing task such a sensitive screening tool.

Because visual and spatial deficits are early signs of dementia, Williams (1992), a geriatrician who co-chairs a national panel to develop guidelines for professionals to screen for dementia, has recommended the task of drawing a clock, set to a specific time, for inclusion in a screening battery. A variety of practitioners who are the first to make contact with the elderly (e.g., nurses, social workers, etc.) could easily learn to administer and interpret clock drawing. Caution, however, should be exercised since absence of evidence is not evidence of absence.

THE TIME SETTING

Clinicians vary as to their use of a time setting in administering the clock-drawing task. In mental-status testing, the task is often administered without specifying any time setting (Strub & Black, 1985). Although it may be of interest to see a patient's spontaneous time setting, there are three shortcomings to this procedure. First, it precludes an assessment of memory for the time setting after the clock features have been drawn. Second, the accuracy with which the clock hands are drawn to represent the setting cannot be evaluated (e.g., whether or not the patient drew the hour and minute hands accurately with regard to an intended target time). Third, specific time settings require the patient to draw one hand on the right and one hand on the left side of the clock face, which affords an assessment of hemi-attentional processing. If a patient with left neglect is allowed to choose his or her own time setting, the patient may spontaneously draw a time that does not have any hands on the left side of space, e.g., "3 o'clock" (the simplest and most common setting), "3:30," or "20 after 2." As a result, the extent of the patient's left neglect may not be appreciated.

For clinicians who specify a time setting when administering a clock-drawing task, the setting used varies greatly. Neurologists commonly require their patients to set the time at "20 after 8." The advantage of this setting is that it requires the patient to draw one hand on each side of the clock, thereby providing an assessment of bilateral hemi-attentional processing. In addition, the hands must be drawn in the inferior visual quadrants, i.e., the "parietal fields." This enhances the sensitivity of the clock-drawing task because the parietal lobes play such an important role in mediating visuoconstruc-tive skills.

Edith Kaplan (Goodglass & Kaplan, 1983; Kaplan, 1988) recommends the use of a "10 after 11" time setting. This setting maintains the advantage of requiring hand placement in both sides of hemispace in the superior quadrants—i.e., the "temporal fields"—and has the added advantage of placing greater demands on executive func-tions mediated by the frontal lobes. Patients with frontal-lobe or diffuse cerebral dysfunction often are impaired in abstract thinking (Goldstein, 1944). Consequently, these patients tend to make "stimulus-bound" errors in which they process information on a more perceptual rather than semantic level. When a patient is instructed to set the hands for "10 after 11," the "10" must be recoded in order to set the minute hand on the number "2." Because a clock includes the number "10" and it is adjacent to the number "11," patients with a tendency to be "captured" (Reason, 1979; Shallice, 1982) or "pulled" to the perceptual features of the command may be prone to make the stimulus-bound error of setting one hand on the "10." In contrast, when representing a time setting such as "20 after 8," the patient, however, must recode the "20" because "20" does not appear on the clock face. Thus, a patient who might have a marked tendency to show a stimulus-bound response is obliged to make the necessary numerical recod-ing if the "20" is to be represented at all.

Some examiners (Spreen and Strauss, 1991) use "20 to 4" as a time setting. This setting differs from "20 after 8" only with regard to the relative proportion of the hands. The only problem with a time setting of "20 to 4" is that an error where both hands are placed on the "4" would be difficult to interpret. For example, was the word "to" confused with "after," were both hands placed on the "4" because of perseveration, or was the underlying problem due to left hemi-inattention?

Of the three most widely used time settings ("10 after 11," "20 after 8," and "3 o'clock"), the most sensitive to neurocognitive dysfunction appears to be the "10 after 11" setting, followed by the "20 after 8" setting, which is not as sensitive to the detection of stimulus-bound tendencies, with the "3 o'clock" setting the least sensitive to verbal command (see Figure 3-7).

DRAWING TO COMMAND AND TO COPY

Although the *command* and *copy* conditions tap overlapping cognitive functions, they differ in important ways. The command condition places relatively greater demand on the language skills needed for comprehension of the verbal instructions, on memory functions needed for both recall of the visual template of a clock and remembering the instructions with regard to the time setting, and on executive functions. As a result, the command condition is especially sensitive to temporal-lobe dysfunction because this region plays an essential role in mediating language (left temporal) and memory processes (right and left temporal), as well as to frontal pathology, which produces deficits in executive function.

In contrast, performance on the copy condition is more dependent on perceptual functions, and thus this condition is especially sensitive to parietal-lobe dysfunction. Patients, therefore, can be selectively impaired on either the command or copy condition, depending on whether their lesions are restricted to temporal or frontal regions on the one hand or parietal regions on the other. A patient with a parietal lesion in the right hemisphere, for example, may draw an acceptable clock to verbal command but omit the numbers in the lower left of a clock drawing to copy. On the other hand, a patient with a right temporal lesion may draw numbers poorly spaced and without a contour to command, whereas the clock drawn to copy is quite adequate (Figure 5-2E, F).

Differences in administration of the clock-drawing task are also notable. Many investigators instruct the subject to "draw the face of a clock, put in all the numbers, and set the time at . . . ." Other investigators do not specify the time until after the clock face and numbers have been drawn. They argue that knowing the time setting in advance of placing the numbers may influence how the subject proceeds. For example, knowing that the time is to be set for "10 after 11," a subject might draw the "11," "12," "1," and "2" in that order, rather than starting with "12" and sequentially drawing the sequence of numbers clockwise; such an atypical response might result in the introduction of errors in spatial organization.

Most clinicians require the patient to produce a freely drawn clock, i.e., the patient is instructed to "draw the face of a clock. . . ." Some investigators (e.g., Wolf-Klein et al., 1989) prefer to present a pre-drawn circle in which the patient would draw in the numbers. One might argue that a patient's circle may not be drawn large enough to contain the numbers, or may not be symmetrical, which might affect the spatial arrangement of the numbers. A reasonable clinical compromise would be to have the patient freely draw the clock face, but to have the examiner provide a pre-drawn circle if the patient produces either no circle, one that is too small, or one that is distorted.

Placement of the clock hands at a given time setting may be constrained by distorted spatial arrangement of the numbers. Thus, presenting the patient with a clock face with numbers permits an assessment of the patient's actual uncontaminated ability to represent a given time.

The above procedures—i.e., the free-drawn, pre-drawn, and examiner clock conditions—represent systematic efforts to parse or isolate some of the major factors involved in the multifactorial cognitive task of clock drawing. The final clock drawing in any one of these conditions, however, may have been achieved by diverse underlying processes that may reflect the activity of distinctly different structures in the central nervous system (Werner, 1937). For Werner (1956), every cognitive act involves "microgenesis" (i.e., "an unfolding process over time"). Thus, a Wernerian, or process-oriented, approach involves close observation and careful monitoring of how a patient proceeds from start to finish.

For example, if a circle (clock contour) is produced, is it drawn counterclockwise (prototypic for right-handers, variable for left-handers)? If, in a right-hander the circle is drawn clockwise, the question of greater dependence on left-hemisphere processing secondary to right-hemisphere dysfunction should be raised. If the circle is too small to write in the numbers, and the patient cannot draw the circle sufficiently larger when requested to, the question of micrographia secondary to a problem in the basal ganglia should be investigated. Does the patient demonstrate good executive skills by organizing the clock face using the numbers "12," "3," "6," and "9" as anchors? Are the numbers correct, but the left side ("11" through "6") written first, and continued counterclockwise (suggesting preference for the left hemi-attentional field contralateral to the right hemisphere and thus a greater reliance on the contribution of the right hemisphere secondary to left-hemisphere dysfunction)? Such observations of the process provides the examiner with a better understanding of impaired as well as spared functions than does a global quantitative score based on a rating of severity of impairment.

Although rating scales or global scores may indeed be suitable for general screening purposes, a process-oriented approach provides finer analyses for hypothesis testing that can yield insights for lateralizing and localizing aspects of performance in the context of current knowledge of brain/behavior relationships. The scoring system presented in the following chapters offers the advantages of both an effective screening tool and a sensitive neuropsychological instrument for analyzing the process by which our patients draw clocks.

2. Normative Study

As noted in the Introduction, clock-drawing tasks have been used to assess the mental status of patients in both neurological and psychiatric settings. Despite the popularity of clock drawing for clinical assessment, the spectrum of clock-drawing ability in neurologically normal individuals has not been formally studied. The interpretation of clock drawings, therefore, has been limited by a lack of normative data. For example, in Chapter 1 we briefly described "stimulus-bound" responses that we and others have observed in patients. Unfortunately, we did not know the base rate of occurrence in neurologically normal individuals. Furthermore, we did not know how and to what extent clock drawing is affected by aging. This is of particular concern when clock drawing is used in elderly patients where it is difficult to separate abnormalities due to neurological dysfunction from changes due to normal aging.

The question of what construct is being measured by clock-drawing tests has never been addressed. Is clock drawing a test of visuospatial or visuoconstructional, praxic, mnemonic, or linguistic abilities? Or, as we suggested in the Introduction, is clock drawing a multifactorial test of all these abilities?

Finally, if a test is to be used as a screening tool, there must be some indication that it is sensitive and specific to neurological dysfunction. Furthermore, the methods used to score the clock drawings should be reliable and stable. Several recent publications have shown that clock-drawing tasks are sensitive measures of cognitive impairment. Rouleau and co-workers (1992) found that patients with Alzheimer's and Huntington's disease were significantly impaired relative to normal controls on clock drawing. Unfortunately, these researchers did not provide measures of sensitivity or specificity. Wolf-Klein et al. (1989) developed a scoring system with a sensitivity of 86.7 percent for Alzheimer's disease and a specificity of 92.7 percent. Sunderland et al. (1989) found that patients with Alzheimer's disease scored significantly lower than did normal controls, but they also did not report measures of sensitivity or specificity. Tuokko et al. (1992) used their scoring system to show that patients with Alzheimer's disease made significantly more errors as compared to normal control subjects, and using a cutoff of more than two errors they reported a sensitivity of 86 percent and a specificity of 92 percent.

As part of the preparation for this book, we developed a brief questionnaire to survey the extent to which professionals use a clock-drawing task as a cognitive measure (see Appendix 1). In February 1989, a total of 595 questionnaires were sent to a selected sample of members of the International Neuropsychological Society and the Behavioral Neurology Society. Three hundred and thirty (55.5%) questionnaires were returned completed. The highest proportion of responses came from the United States (66.5%, primarily Massachusetts, New York, California, and Florida), from Canada (15.2%), and from Great Britain (4.4%). Other countries represented were Italy, Australia, Netherlands, Denmark, Israel, Norway, and Sweden. Respondents were primarily neurologists and neuropsychologists who were asked to indicate (1) whether or not they used a clock-drawing task in their clinical practice and/or in their research; (2) how many years they had been using this task; (3) how they had first learned about clock drawing; (4) how useful they felt clock drawing to be; and (5) details of their administration.

Sixty-three percent of the respondents indicated they used a clock-drawing task. Of those who used this task, 98 percent employed it in their clinical practice and 40 percent used it in their research. The mean number of years that clock drawing was used in clinical practice was 10.74 (ranging from 0.30 to 40 years), and the mean number of years clock drawing was used in research was 7.94 (ranging from 0.50 to 40 years).

Respondents indicated that they had first learned about clock drawing as a cognitive measure from a variety of sources. Approximately 62 percent had first learned of the procedure from a specific individual. Approximately 48 percent first learned of clock drawing from a neuropsychologist. The most commonly cited neuropsychologists were Arthur Benton, Dean Delis, Edith Kaplan, and Ralph Reitan. Approximately 20 percent first learned of clock drawing from a neurologist. The most commonly cited neurologists were MacDonald Critchley, Norman Geschwind, Henri Hécaen, and Kenneth Heilman. Twenty-one percent of respondents first learned of clock drawing from the literature. The most frequent book cited was *Higher Cortical Functions in Man,* by A. R. Luria. Other texts cited were *The Parietal Lobes,* by MacDonald Critchley; *The Assessment of Aphasia and Related Disorders,* by Goodglass and Kaplan; *Aphasia and Kindred Disorders of Speech,* by Henry Head; *Human Neuropsychology,* by Hécaen and Albert; *Clinical Neuropsychology,* by Heilman and Valenstein; *Neuropsychological Assessment,* by Lezak; *The Mental Status Examination in Neurology,* by Strub and Black; and an article "Visual-Spatial Neglect Subsequent to Brain Injury," by La Pointe and Culton (*Journal of Speech and Hearing Disorders, 1969*).

Respondents rated how useful they felt clock drawing to be on a scale from 1 to 5 (5 being most useful). Approximately 90 percent found it useful in the screening of cognitive impairment (mean rating was 3.91). The same number found it useful in monitoring the course of cognitive deficits over time (mean rating was 3.27). Forty-six percent found clock drawing useful in research, but less so than in clinical practice (mean rating was 2.94).

More users of the clock-drawing task asked their patients to draw a clock freely (83%) than to set the time on a pre-drawn clock (40%), or to copy a clock (39%). Of those respondents who asked their patients to draw a clock freely, 91 percent had them put the numbers on the clock, and 84 percent had them set the time. The task of copying a clock or setting the time on a pre-drawn clock was usually administered only when a patient exhibited difficulty in freely drawing a clock. The time setting most frequently used was "10 after 11" (44% for the freely drawn clock, 26% for the pre-drawn clock, and 50% for the clock copy). Other time settings that were requested were "3 o'clock," and "20 after 8," and less frequently "9 o'clock," "10 past 10," "10 to 11," "9:15," "7:30," "1:00," and "10 to 9."

Results of this survey indicate that a clock-drawing task is frequently used throughout the world in the assessment of cognitive deficits in brain-injured patients. Although it has been used for years in both clinical practice and research, many of the respondents expressed a need for the development of a standardized method of administration and scoring of the clock-drawing task.

To address the lack of normative data and to determine construct validity we examined clock-drawing ability along with several tests of neuropsychological functions in a large sample of neurologically normal individuals ranging in age from 20 to 90 years. To evaluate the clinical sensitivity and specificity, we compared the clock drawings of normal elderly subjects to the drawings of patients with Alzheimer's disease. We included three basic clock-drawing conditions in our normative study that varied from unstructured to highly structured.

In the free-drawn condition, the subjects were requested to draw all aspects of a clock, including the contour, numbers, and hands and to set the hands at a specified time. In the pre-drawn condition, a pre-drawn contour was provided and the subjects were asked to reproduce the numbers and hands and to set the clock hands at a specified time. In the examiner clock condition, a pre-drawn contour with numbers was provided and the subjects were requested only to set the hands at a specified time. The free-drawn condition contains all of the elements of the clock-drawing task including contour, numbers, hands, and center. At face value, the free-drawn condition appears to represent a visuoconstructional task because the subjects must reproduce visual aspects of a clock without a model to copy.

The pre-drawn condition was similar except that the general framework (e.g., the contour) was provided. The examiner clock evaluated knowledge of the concept of time as represented in a familiar, analog format. The examiner clock controlled for variations in the size and shape of the clock face, as well as the sequencing and placement of the numbers, the greatest emphasis being placed on the placement of the hands at the appropriate position of the clock face. For example, the knowledge implicit in placing the hands on a clock at "10 after 11" is that 10 minutes after the hour is represented by the digit "2," the hour is represented by the digit "11," and the minute hand is longer than the hour hand.

In the free-drawn condition, subjects were presented with a blank sheet of $8^{1}/_{2}$-by-11-inch paper and given the following instructions: "I would like you to draw a clock and put in the numbers." After completing this task, the patient was given the following instructions: "Now I would like you to set the time at a quarter to seven." In the pre-drawn condition, subjects were given a sheet of $8^{1}/_{2}$-by-11-inch paper with a circle 11.7 cm ($4^{5}/_{8}$ in) in diameter and instructed to "Put the numbers on the clock and set the time at 5 after 6." In the examiner clock condition, subjects were given three sheets of paper with 11.7-cm (4⅝ in) circles containing the numbers 1 to 12 and asked to set the times at "20 after 8," "10 after 11," and "3 o'clock," respectively. The three conditions were presented in a fixed order as follows: free-drawn, pre-drawn, and examiner clocks.

A comprehensive list of descriptors of responses was prepared on the basis of past experience with clock drawings and a consideration of possible and likely responses. The number of items varied for each condition because of the different aspects of the clocks that subjects were required to draw. In the scoring of free-drawn clocks, the drawings were analyzed according to the broad categories of contour, numbers, hands, and center. Scoring of the pre-drawn clock was based on the categories of numbers, hands, and center. Examiner clocks were scored only on the categories of hands and center. The complete list of descriptors is provided in Appendix 2.

A total of 348 subjects ranging in age from 20 to 90 years participated in the clock-drawing tasks. All subjects were volunteers recruited through advertisements in local newspapers and radio shows, at senior citizen centers, and in various community centers in the Metropolitan Toronto area. All met the following inclusion criteria: (1) English was their first language; (2) no history of alcoholism; (3) no history of depression or other psychiatric disorder; (4) no history of stroke, transient ischemic attacks, or seizures; (5) no history of head injury resulting in loss of consciousness lasting longer than one minute, and (6) no subjective memory complaints. The subject pool was subdivided into seven age groups by decades: 20–29, 30–39, 40–49, 50–59, 60–69, 70–79, and 80+ years of age. A description of the respective age groups in terms of sex, age, education, and handedness is given in Table 2-1.

Following the initial scoring of all clocks, the data were analyzed to determine which responses were present at a high or low rate, respectively. A subset of descriptors was selected if they occurred, or did not occur, in at least 90 percent of subjects in the youngest age group. This list of descriptors was evaluated by the authors to determine which were considered characteristic of a "good" or "bad" clock. The definition of a "good" or "bad" clock was determined upon consensus. The following question was asked for each item: "Would the presence or absence of this item in anyway contribute significantly to a 'good' or 'bad' clock?" For example, the normative data indicated that at least 90 percent of all subjects who drew "arrowheads"

TABLE 2-1. Profile of Subjects, by Age Group

	20–29	30–39	40–49	50–59	60–69	70–79	80–90
N	40	40	40	52	76	59	41
Mean Age (years)	24.4	34.4	44.6	54.9	64.6	74.2	82.4
Mean Education (years)	15.3	15.3	16.3	15.3	13.8	13.7	13.1
Male	19	21	21	22	30	24	17
Female	21	19	19	30	46	35	24
Handedness							
right	37	29	38	41	65	53	36
left	1	6	1	9	4	3	0
ambidextrous	2	5	1	2	7	3	5

TABLE 2-2. 6:45 Free-drawn Clock: Percentage of Subjects with a Given Response, by Age Group

	20–29	30–39	40–49	50–59	60–69	70–79	80–90
N	40	40	39	52	75	54	41
Contour:							
Acceptable contour drawn	100.0	100.0	100.0	100.0	100.0	100.0	100.0
Contour is not too small nor overdrawn nor reproduced repeatedly	100.0	100.0	100.0	100.0	100.0	100.0	92.7
Numbers:							
Only numbers 1–12 (without adding extra numbers or omitting numbers)	97.5	97.5	100.0	96.2	97.4	92.5	95.1
Arabic number representation	95.0	97.5	97.4	98.1	97.3	100.0	87.8
Numbers written in the correct order	100.0	100.0	100.0	100.0	100.0	100.0	100.0
Paper not rotated while drawing numbers	100.0	100.0	100.0	100.0	100.0	90.7	90.2
Numbers in the correct position	97.5	100.0	97.4	96.2	82.7	72.2	75.6
All numbers located inside contour	90.0	97.5	94.9	90.4	94.7	92.6	90.2
Hands:							
Clock has 2 hands/or marks	100.0	100.0	100.0	100.0	100.0	90.8	90.3
Hour target number indicated in some manner	97.5	97.5	100.0	96.2	94.7	100.0	92.7
Minute target number indicated in some manner	100.0	100.0	100.0	98.1	93.3	88.9	82.9
Hands in correct proportion (minute hand longer)	95.0	87.5	89.7	78.8	77.3	66.7	65.9
No superfluous markings	97.5	97.5	97.4	96.2	90.7	87.0	87.8
Hands are joined or within 12 mm ($^1/_2$ in) of joining	100.0	100.0	100.0	100.0	100.0	95.9	100.0
Center:							
Clock has a center (drawn or inferred/ extrapolated at the point where 2 hands meet)	100.0	100.0	100.0	100.0	100.0	92.5	92.7

6:05 Pre-drawn Clock: Percentage of Subjects with a Given Response, by Age Group

	20–29	30–39	40–49	50–59	60–69	70–79	80–90
N	40	40	39	52	76	59	41
Numbers:							
Only numbers 1–12 (without adding extra numbers of omitting numbers)	100.0	100.0	92.3	94.2	94.8	91.5	90.2
Arabic number representation	92.5	100.0	97.4	96.2	97.4	100.0	87.8
Numbers written in the correct order	100.0	100.0	100.0	100.0	100.0	100.0	97.6
Paper not rotated while drawing numbers	100.0	100.0	100.0	100.0	100.0	93.2	87.8
Numbers in correct position	97.5	95.0	92.3	98.1	86.8	74.6	63.4
All numbers located inside contour	90.0	97.5	92.3	92.3	93.4	93.2	87.8
Hands:							
Clock has 2 hands/or marks	100.0	100.0	100.0	100.0	100.0	89.9	90.3
Hour target number indicated in some manner	100.0	100.0	100.0	100.0	100.0	100.0	100.0
Minute target number indicated in some manner	100.0	100.0	100.0	96.2	98.7	88.1	87.8

(continued)

TABLE 2-2. 6:05 Pre-drawn Clock *(Continued)*

	20–29	30–39	40–49	50–59	60–69	70–79	80–90
Hands in correct proportion (minute hand longer)	92.5	85.0	89.7	80.8	73.7	50.8	51.2
No superfluous markings	100.0	97.5	92.3	96.2	97.4	89.8	92.7
Hands are joined or within 12 mm (¹/₂ in) of joining	100.0	95.0	100.0	100.0	97.4	94.3	100.0
Center:							
Clock has a center (drawn or inferred/ extrapolated at the point where 2 hands meet)	100.0	100.0	100.0	100.0	97.4	89.8	95.1

11:10 Examiner Clock: Percentage of Subjects with a Given Response, by Age Group

N	40	40	40	52	76	59	41
Hands:							
Clock has 2 hands/or marks	100.0	97.5	100.0	100.0	98.7	91.5	87.8
Hour target number indicated in some manner	100.0	97.5	100.0	100.0	98.7	100.0	100.0
Minute target indicated in some manner	100.0	100.0	100.0	96.2	100.0	88.1	90.2
Hands in correct proportion (minute hand longer)	97.5	90.0	100.0	86.5	82.9	74.6	53.7
Hour hand/mark is displaced from hour target number within limits set by normative data (−6 to 10 degrees)	97.5	95.0	92.5	90.4	97.5	91.5	78.0
Minute hand/mark is displaced from minute number within limits set by normative data (−3 to 6 degrees)	100.0	100.0	92.5	98.1	98.7	83.9	70.2
No superfluous markings on the clock	100.0	97.5	95.0	100.0	94.7	94.9	100.0
Hands are joined or within 12 mm (¹/₂ in) of joining	100.0	97.4	100.0	98.1	98.7	94.4	100.0
Center:							
Clock has a center (drawn or inferred/ extrapolated at the point where 2 hands meet)	100.0	95.0	100.0	100.0	98.4	86.4	90.2
Center is displaced from the vertical axis within 5.0 mm (³/₁₆ in) to the right or left of the axis	95.0	94.7	97.5	100.0	97.3	94.1	89.2
Center is displaced from the horizontal axis within 5.0 mm (³/₁₆ in) below the axis or 7.0 mm (⁵/₁₆ in) above the axis	97.5	89.5	90.0	94.2	90.7	92.2	91.9

8:20 Examiner Clock: Percentage of Subjects with a Given Response, by Age Group

N	40	40	40	52	76	59	41
Hands:							
Clock has 2 hands/or marks	100.0	100.0	100.0	100.0	100.0	91.5	87.8
Hour target number indicated in some manner	100.0	100.0	100.0	100.0	100.0	100.0	100.0

(continued)

TABLE 2-2. 8:20 Examiner Clock *(Continued)*

	20–29	30–39	40–49	50–59	60–69	70–79	80–90
Minute target number indicated in some manner	100.0	97.5	100.0	98.1	98.7	91.5	90.2
Hands in correct proportion (minute hand longer)	92.5	90.0	90.0	88.5	78.9	69.5	68.3
Hour hand/mark is displaced from hour target number within limits set by normative data (−3 to 15 degrees)	95.0	90.0	97.5	96.2	98.7	98.3	100.0
Minute hand/mark is displaced from minute number within limits set by normative data (−6 to 3 degrees)	95.0	95.0	92.5	96.1	90.7	87.5	83.8
No superfluous markings on the clock	100.0	100.0	95.0	100.0	100.0	98.3	90.2
Hands are joined or within 12 mm (¹/₂ in) of joining	100.0	100.0	100.0	100.0	98.7	96.3	100.0
Center:							
Clock has a center (drawn or inferred/ extrapolated at the point where 2 hands meet)	100.0	100.0	97.5	100.0	98.7	88.1	92.7
Center is displaced from the vertical axis within 5.0 mm (³/₁₆ in) to the right or left of the axis	97.5	97.5	95.0	96.2	93.4	92.3	100.0
Center is displaced from the horizontal axis within 5.0 mm (³/₁₆ in) below the axis or 7.0 mm (⁵/₁₆) above the axis	95.0	90.0	95.0	96.2	92.1	90.4	94.7

3:00 Examiner Clock: Percentage of Subjects with a Given Response, by Age Group

N	40	40	40	52	76	59	41
Hands:							
Clock has 2 hands/or marks	100.0	100.0	100.0	100.0	100.0	91.5	87.8
Hour target number indicated in some manner	100.0	100.0	100.0	100.0	100.0	100.0	100.0
Minute target number indicated in some manner	100.0	100.0	100.0	100.0	100.0	96.6	92.7
Hands in correct proportion (minute hand longer)	95.0	85.0	87.5	84.6	84.2	62.7	53.7
Hour hand/mark is displaced from hour target number within limits set by normative data (−3 to 3 degrees)	90.0	90.0	97.5	100.0	96.1	96.6	97.6
Minute hand/mark is displaced from minute number within limits set by normative data (−3 to 3 degrees)	100.0	97.5	87.5	96.2	94.7	89.5	97.4
No superfluous markings on the clock	97.5	97.5	95.0	100.0	98.7	100.0	97.6
Hands are joined or within 12 mm (¹/₂ in) of joining	100.0	100.0	100.0	100.0	98.7	96.3	97.2
Center:							
Clock has a center (drawn or inferred/ extrapolated at the point where 2 hands meet)	100.0	100.0	100.0	100.0	98.7	88.1	92.7

(continued)

TABLE 2-2.   *(Continued)*

	20–29	30–39	40–49	50–59	60–69	70–79	80–90
Center is displaced from the vertical axis within 5.0 mm (³/₁₆ in) to the right or left of the axis	100.0	95.0	100.0	94.2	90.8	96.2	92.1
Center is displaced from the horizontal axis within 5.0 mm (³/₁₆ in) below the axis or 7.0 mm (⁵/₁₆ in) above the axis	100.0	95.0	100.0	98.1	98.7	96.2	97.4

placed them on both hands—that is, 10 percent or less drew only one arrowhead on either the minute hand or the hour hand. By consensus, however, we decided that although drawing only one arrowhead was unusual it was not considered as contributing significantly to a "bad" clock. This item was, therefore, not defined as a critical item.

The smaller subset of descriptors was then used to establish a set of "critical items" from which an objective scoring procedure could be developed. Details of the items chosen and their probability of occurrence for each clock condition in the normative study are presented in Table 2-2. The free-drawn clock condition consisted of 15 critical items that constituted a total score of 15. In addition, items were grouped according to those relating to the contour (2 items), numbers (6 items), hands (6 items), and center (1 item). The pre-drawn clock condition consisted of 13 critical items grouped according to numbers (6 items), hands (6 items), and center (1 item). The examiner clock condition consisted of 11 critical items grouped according to hands (8 items) and center (3 items).

Clock Drawing in Normals

All subjects in each age group were capable of drawing an acceptable contour in the free-drawn condition. The definition of "acceptable" was any closed contour. Closure was considered adequate if the line(s) used to define the contour were touching or overlapping. There was a wide range in shape and symmetry, as illustrated in Figure 2-1.

The vast majority of clocks tended to be circular or oval in shape although some were square, rectangular, or octagonal. One contour was even heart-shaped (Figure 2-1C). Some clocks contained various fanciful elaborations such as cases, bells, or legs (Figure 2-1D).

The size of the contour in the free-drawn condition showed considerable variation. The size was considered unacceptable only if it was not possible to include all numbers and hands within the contour. A comparison of the relative clock sizes is shown in Figure 2-2. Although some small clocks occurred in all age groups, they were unacceptably small in only three cases in the oldest age group (see Figure 2-3). Figure 2-3A illustrates the clock of an 88-year-old subject who drew a contour that was too small despite

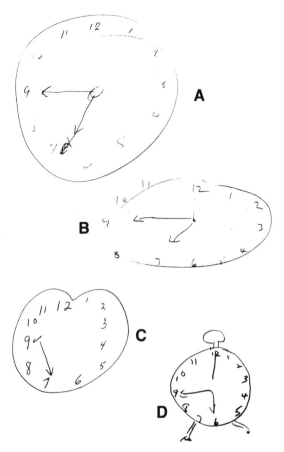

Figure 2–1 Examples of acceptable contours. (A) 70-year-old male. (B) 52-year-old male. (C) 65-year-old female. (D) Example of acceptable coutour with elaboration of nonessential details: alarm clock with bell, legs, and second hand; 79-year-old male.

two attempts. Figure 2-3B shows the attempts of an 80-year-old subject who made the clock face too small to include the hands.

The vast majority of subjects across all age groups used Arabic as opposed to Roman numerals in both the free-drawn and pre-drawn conditions. A clock with Roman numerals, however, is illustrated in Figure 2-4. Two features peculiar to timepieces with Roman numerals should be mentioned. First, it is customary for the Roman numerals to be oriented in a radial fashion with the base of each numeral facing the center of the clock. Therefore, the numerals appear upright from the perspective of someone standing at the center of the clock. Second, the numeral "4" is represented as "IIII" rather than "IV." Although these customs appear to be observed on almost every clock or watch we were able to find, few people, except perhaps watchmakers, appear to be cognizant of them. Therefore, in scoring clocks with Roman numerals we

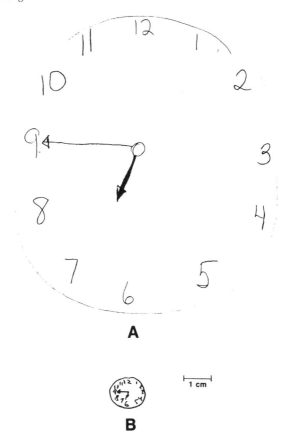

A

B

Figure 2–2   Examples of acceptable clock contour size. (A) Largest clock; 22-year-old male. (B) Example of worst acceptable case; 46-year-old male.

accepted both "IIII" and "IV" for the number "4." We also allowed Roman numerals to be oriented the customary way, such as an upside down "VI," or in the usual upright orientation for Arabic numerals. It is interesting to note that the subject who drew the clocks in Figure 2-4 had difficulty deciding how to represent the number "4." In the free-drawn clock, this subject wrote "III" for "3," "IIII" for "4," and then continued in the response set to write "IIIII" for "5" and "IIIIII" for "6"!

Ninety percent or more of the subjects across all ages placed the numbers 1 to 12 on their clocks without omissions or additions. There was no apparent difference in this capacity in either free-drawn or pre-drawn clock conditions. Errors in this category included the simple omission of one or more numbers (Figure 2-5A), the omission of a number with the perseveration of another number (Figure 2-5B), or repeating one or more numbers (Figure 2-5C). The worst case of omission and adding of numbers is illustrated by the clock drawn by a 77-year-old subject in Figure 2-6A and 2-6B. This subject placed only the numbers 1 through 6 on the first attempt of the free-drawn clock

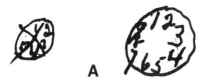

A

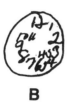

B

Figure 2–3   Examples of clocks too small to contain all numbers and hands. (A) No hands and only numbers 1 through 9 present; 88-year-old male. (B) All numbers present but no hands; 80-year-old female.

but on the second attempt wrote the numbers "12" and "6" and then placed the numerals "5–60" at the remaining 5-minute intervals. On the pre-drawn clock, the same subject wrote the number "12" followed by the numbers "5–55" (in increments of 5). Only one subject failed to place all numbers in the correct sequence (Figure 2-7). This was an 86-year-old subject who placed the numbers in a counterclockwise sequence.

   Subjects tended not to rotate the paper as they wrote the numbers. Rotating the paper occurred only in the 70–79 and 80+ age groups and was seen in about 10 percent of the subjects in these age categories. Rotation of the paper should, therefore, not be considered pathological. Rotating the paper, however, typically resulted in numbers being poorly oriented. Examples of rotation by a 75-year-old subject are illustrated in Figure 2-8.

   Numbers were considered to be placed correctly as long as they were put in a position that would not normally be occupied by another number. For example, all numbers in the clocks in Figures 2-1 and 2-2 were considered to be placed correctly. The numbers of the clock in Figure 2-3B were considered to be placed incorrectly because the numeral "11" was placed near the center due to size restrictions. Figure 2-5B, on the other hand, illustrates a case where a second number "10" was placed

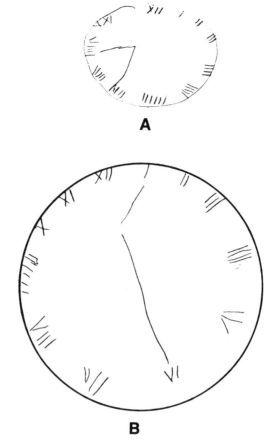

A

B

Figure 2–4   Only Roman spoken here! Examples of clocks with Roman numerals. (A) and (B) 84-year-old female. Note representation of numerals 5 through 9 in (A) and absence of numeral 5 in (B).

where the number "11" should be situated. This was not scored as a number being placed in the incorrect position, because a "10" was already in the correct position, but only as a simple omission with substitution. Compare this with Figure 2-5A where the number "1" was omitted and the number "2" was also placed in the incorrect position. The "2" was scored as being incorrectly placed. Figure 2-9A is an example of the worst allowable placement of numbers and occurred in a 53-year-old subject. Figure 2-9B is another example in which one or more numbers were scored as being incorrectly placed. Examples of poor number placement occurred in all age groups but was most frequently seen in subjects over the age of 59.

Subjects tended to place all numbers within the contours of the clock in both the free-drawn and pre-drawn conditions. The frequency of either all or a portion of the numbers being placed outside the contours was approximately equivalent across all age

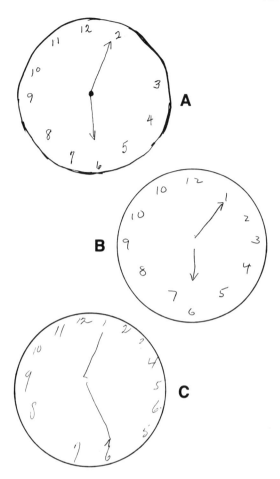

Figure 2–5 Examples of omission or addition of numbers. (A) Omission of number 1 and misplacement of number 2; 83-year-old female. (B) Omission of number 11 with perseveration of number 10; 65-year-old male. (C) Addition of extra numbers 5 and 6; 70-year-old female.

groups. Figure 2-9C shows a representative case of numbers being placed outside the contour. In the case illustrated, all other aspects of the clock were considered correct.

Of all features of a clock, the hands are most critical for representing time. Numbers or marks may help to indicate precisely the minute or hour, but it is only by using the relative positions and proportions of the hands as cues that time can be estimated to within a 5-minute interval of the actual time. It is relatively common for timepieces not to have either numerals or any indication of the minutes. In fact, very expensive timepieces often lack numbers. The distinction between the hour and minute hands was based upon an arbitrary decision dating back many centuries. We all learn at an early age that the "big hand" represents the minutes and the "little hand" represents the

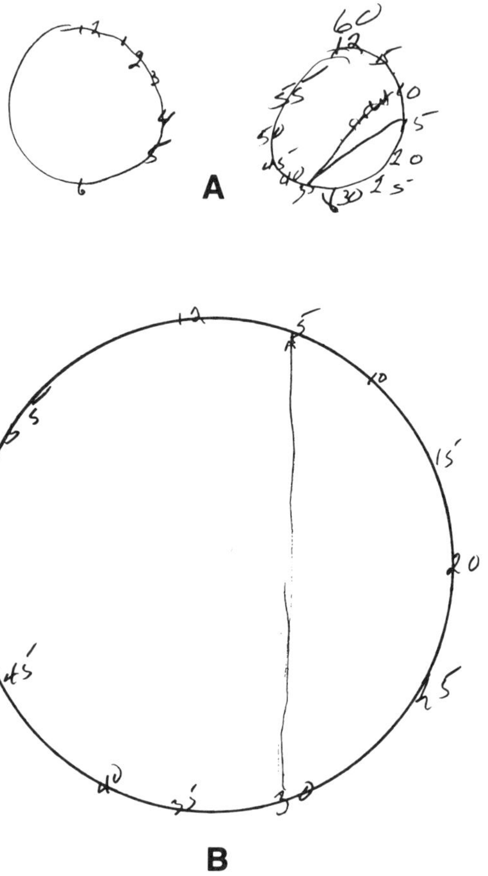

Figure 2–6 (A) and (B) Omission and substitution of numbers; 77-year-old female.

hours. Once this rule and the relative placement of the numbers are learned, time can be decoded with a glance at the positions of the hands.

The greatest difficulty that the numbers pose is their dual representation of hours as well as minutes. The hour representation is straightforward (and concrete), but the minute representation is for the most part ambiguous and abstract. For example, the numeral "1" can represent "5 minutes past the hour" or "5 after the hour" or "00:05." The only example where the numeral and minute are directly translatable is the numeral "10" for "10 minutes to the hour." Even in the latter case, however, "10" can also represent "50 minutes past the hour." Because the distinction between the minute and hour hands is arbitrary and the representation of minutes is ambiguous, it is not surprising that the most frequent errors across all three conditions involved these two features.

The scoring system took into account indication of the hour and minutes in some

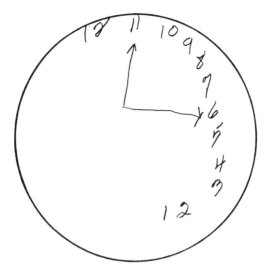

Figure 2–7   Example of improper sequencing of numbers; 86-year-old female.

manner other than by the use of conventional hands. Ninety-two percent or more of the subjects at all ages were able to indicate the hour target number correctly in some manner in all clock conditions. The ability to indicate the minute number was more variable. The greatest number of errors occurred in the 70–79 and 80+ age groups.

Examples of how time can be indicated without the use of hands are given in Figure 2-10. Figure 2-10A is a pre-drawn clock where a tick, or check mark, was placed next to the target numbers for both the hour and the minute. Figure 2-10B is an examiner clock of another subject who used a short line segment next to the target number for the hour. The subject failed to place any mark next to the minute number, however. Figure 2-11 gives examples of clocks in which target numbers were marked by hands that were joined well off center or by hands that failed to be joined. Figures 2-11A and 2-11B are a single subject's pre-drawn and examiner clocks where the hands emanate from a point near the contour although the hour and minutes are both accurately marked. Figure 2-11C is another subject's examiner clock in which both the hour and minutes are accurately marked by short line segments, which if extended would join near the actual center. Notice also that in Figure 2-11C arrowheads were placed on both hands but they point toward the center rather than toward the periphery of the clock.

Owing to variations in clock shape, size, and number of placements in both the free-drawn and pre-drawn condition, it was not possible to define the degree of precision by which subjects were able to place hands or marks near the hour or minute numbers. The examiner clocks, however, provided a means of assessing the placement of hands or marks. Table 2-2 shows the percentage of normal subjects who placed a hand or mark within the limits set by the normative data for each of the different time settings. Superficially, it would appear that the wider degree of latitude for the hour as opposed

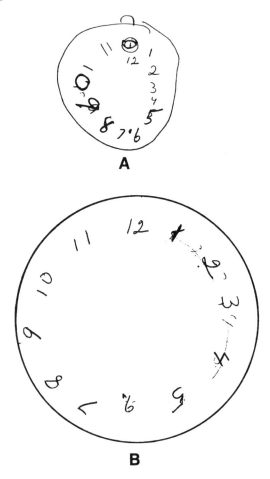

A

B

Figure 2–8   Examples of rotation of paper while drawing resulting in numbers being misoriented; (A) and (B) 75-year-old female.

to the minute number contradicts our earlier statement that it is more difficult to place the minute hand correctly. In all clocks, however, subjects were required to place the minute hand/mark at a specific numeral, because all times used fell at the discrete 5-minute intervals. The hour hand, however, must be displaced slightly off the target number for all times requested, except for 3 o'clock, to be accurately represented. Therefore, the greater variability in hour hand/mark placement likely reflects subjects' attempts to represent accurately this displacement rather than an error in indicating the hour.

Accurate representation of the relative proportion of the hand size was the most common difficulty encountered. Hands were considered to be proportioned correctly if the hour hand was perceptibly or measurably shorter than the minute hand. Errors in proportion occurred in all age groups but increased in frequency with age. Figure

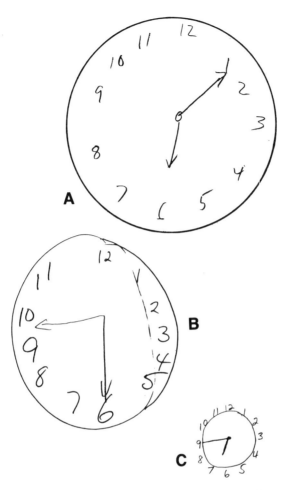

Figure 2–9   Examples of good and poor placement of numbers. (A) Illustration of worst allowable case of proper placement of numbers; 53-year-old male. (B) Improper placement of numbers 10 and 11; 35-year-old male. (C) Example of placement of numbers outside clock contour; 25-year-old male.

2-12A illustrates a case where the minute hand is just perceptibly longer than the hour hand, and Figure 2-12B shows a case where the minute hand is shorter than the hour hand.

Eighty-nine percent or more of the subjects across all age groups were able to place the intersection of the hands within 5 mm (³/₁₆ in) to the right or left of center and 5 mm above or 7 mm (⁵/₁₆ in) below center on the examiner clocks. In cases where the hands did not physically touch or intersect, an extrapolated center was approximated by extending the subject's hands to a point of intersection. In a few clocks (Figure 2-11A and 2-11B) the hands were joined near the periphery.

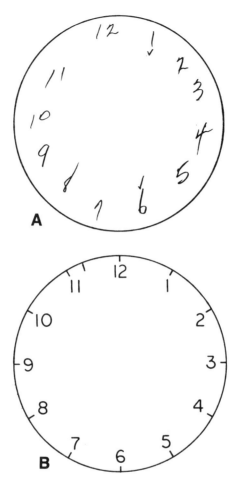

Figure 2–10   Examples of time being indicated by some means other than hands. (A) Target numbers indicated by marks next to 1 and 6 for 6:05; 78-year-old female. (B) Hour target number indicated by short mark between 11 and 12 but minute not indicated; 73-year-old male.

Ninety percent or more of all subjects drew two hands on their clocks except in four conditions. The exceptions occurred in the 70–79-year-old group in the pre-drawn condition (89.9%), and the 80+ group for all three examiner clocks (87.8%). In those cases where only one hand was drawn, the most common occurrence was for a single hand to be drawn between the two target numbers, as illustrated in Figure 2-13. In all cases, both target numbers were indicated and the marks were within the limitations for precision of placement described above.

Many subjects failed to join the hands completely (if two hands were drawn) but 90 percent or more of the subjects brought the hands within 12 mm (½ in) of joining.

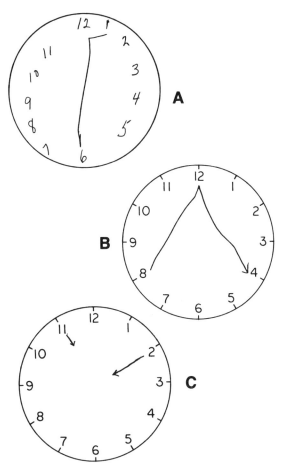

Figure 2–11   Examples of target numbers being indicated by "hand-like" marks. (A) and (B) Hands join well off center but endpoints are positioned near target numbers; 70-year-old female. (C) Hour and minute accurately marked by short line segments; 78-year-old female.

Very few subjects placed superfluous hands or marks on the clock face. Marks that were clearly intended to represent either 1- or 5-minute intervals were not considered superfluous (our own examiner clocks had marks at the 5-minute intervals). There was one case, however, where marks placed at the 5-minute intervals were defined as superfluous. Figures 2-14A and 2-14B illustrate interval marks that were extended to the center to form a "spokes-of-the-wheel" configuration. This was considered super-fluous because the minute marks do not typically extend to the center. One common "superfluous" mark may have represented attempts at placing a second hand (Figure 2-15A). An unusual case of superfluous markings is illustrated in Figure 2-15B where a "Christmas tree" pattern was produced. In Figure 2-15B the time is simply written as

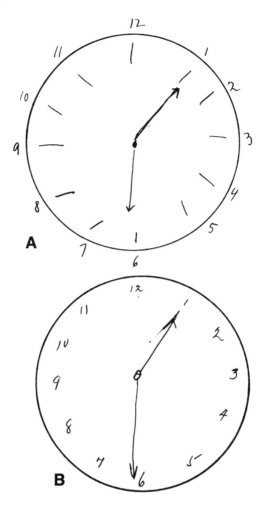

Figure 2–12 Examples of relative proportion of hour and minute hands. (A) Minute hand is just perceptibly longer than hour hand; 68-year-old female. (B) Hour hand is perceptibly longer than minute hand; 81-year-old male.

"605" next to the number "6" in a literal fashion. Figures 2-15C and 2-15D illustrate a very uncommon occurrence among the normal subjects that was only found in the three oldest age groups. In both cases, the subject wrote the number "10" after the "11" and the number "20" after the "8" for "10 after 11" and "20 after 8," respectively. This error represents a concrete interpretation of the instructions and is suggestive of frontal system dysfunction. A variation of this stimulus-bound behavior is illustrated in Figure 2-16A where the minute hand is placed at the "5" instead of the "1" for "5 after 6." Another example of stimulus-bound behavior is illustrated in Figure 2-16B. Here the

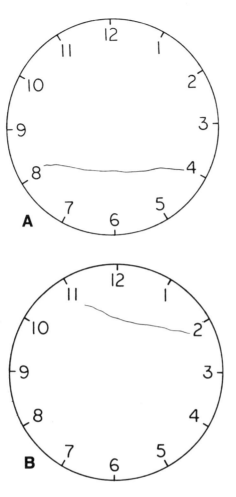

Figure 2–13 Examples of single-handed clocks. (A) and (B) Hour and minute numbers indicated by single hand; 77-year-old female.

subject was asked to set the time at "a quarter to 7." Apparently the subject decoded the time as "6:45" but then placed hands at the numbers "6," "4," and "5"!

Analysis of Total Clock Scores

The means for the total scores for each clock condition are listed by age group in Table 2-3. The ANOVA indicated a significant main effect for age for the total score for all conditions ($p < .0001$). A Newman-Keuls test revealed that the mean total scores for

A

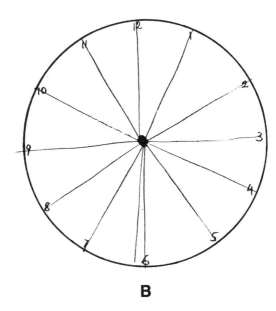

B

Figure 2–14   Examples of superfluous marks or hands. (A) and (B) "spokes of a wheel" configuration; 73-year-old male.

both the 70–79 and 80+ age groups were significantly different from all other age groups but not from each other ($p < .05$).

Table 2-4 presents the cumulative frequencies and percentile rankings for the total clock scores for each age group. The effect of age on the total clock scores is evident in the range of scores for age groups; the greatest ranges occur at the 70–79 and 80+ age groups.

Reliability among three raters was found to be very high using our "critical item" scoring system. The Pearson correlation coefficients for the various conditions were as follows: Free-drawn, $r = .989, .813, .790$ (all $p < .001$); mean $= .865$. Pre-drawn, $r = .838, .840, .845$ (all $p < .001$); mean $= .841$. Examiner clock, $r = .629, .716, .740$ (all $p < .001$); mean $= .695$.

Test-retest reliability as measured by Spearman rank-order correlations were very low and insignificant except for one condition, the examiner clock at "11:10" ($r =$

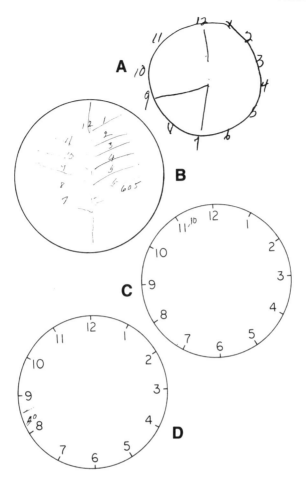

Figure 2–15   Examples of superfluous marks or hands. (A) Superfluous mark representing a second hand; 74-year-old male. (B) "Christmas tree"; 81-year-old female. (C) and (D) Minutes indicated as a concrete interpretation for 11:10 (C) and 8:20 (D); 81-year-old female.

.9377, $p < .02$). This apparent lack of reliability reflects the restricted range of scores across the various conditions. The only significant correlation was obtained on the condition that also had the greatest range in scores. Scores remained relatively stable across the two administrations except for the pre-drawn condition; on retest the subjects tended to obtain higher scores (Sign Test; $p = .0352$) for the pre-drawn clock, but no other test-retest differences were significant.

To determine what neuropsychological abilities are related to clock drawing we administered the following neuropsychological battery to 171 normal subjects: (1) an abbreviated version of the Revised Wechsler Adult Intelligence Scale (WAIS-R) consisting of the Information, Picture Completion, Block Design, Vocabulary, and Arith-

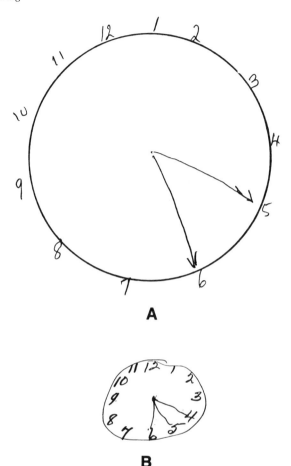

A

B

Figure 2–16   Examples of "stimulus pull." (A) Time set at "5 after 6," note minute hand set at number 5 instead of 1; 82-year-old male. (B) Time set at "quarter to seven"; note two hands at 4 and 5 in an attempt to represent 6:45; 80-year-old female.

metic subtests (Wechsler, 1981); (2) the Wisconsin Card Sorting Test (WCST) (Heaton, 1981); (3) Controlled Word Association (FAS) Test (Benton & des Hamsher, 1989); and (4) the Rey-Osterrieth Complex Figure (Rey, 1941) consisting of copy, immediate, and 50-minute delayed reproduction from memory conditions. The tests provided measures of general intellectual functioning, long-term memory, concept formation, inductive reasoning, mental flexibility and verbal, visuoperceptual, and visuoconstructional abilities.

Total scores for each clock were correlated with all other clock drawings as well as scores on various neuropsychological tests. The total clock drawing scores are intercorrelated, although in most cases the intercorrelations between the clock scores are no

TABLE 2-3. Total Clock Scores

Clock Condition		Age Group						
		20–29	30–39	40–49	50–59	60–69	70–79	80–90
6:45 Free-Drawn	Mean	14.70	14.75	14.77	14.50	14.28	13.68	13.34
	SD	.61	.49	.43	.83	.88	1.84	2.09
6:05 Pre-Drawn	Mean	12.72	12.70	12.56	12.54	12.38	11.46	11.22
	SD	.50	.56	.94	.73	.80	1.55	1.93
11:10 Examiner	Mean	10.80	10.42	10.68	10.60	10.53	9.54	9.34
	SD	.40	1.52	.62	.69	.90	2.24	2.38
8:20 Examiner	Mean	10.75	10.60	10.65	10.71	10.51	9.69	9.71
	SD	.44	.81	.62	.57	.68	2.20	2.18
3:00 Examiner	Mean	10.82	10.60	10.68	10.73	10.60	9.80	9.73
	SD	.38	.54	.57	.53	.63	1.96	2.05

higher than intercorrelations with other tests of visuoconstructional abilities such as the WAIS-R Block Design or scores from the Rey-Osterrieth Complex Figure (see Table 2-5).

Total clock scores for each clock-drawing condition, along with selected neuropsychological test scores, were analyzed by a principal components analysis followed by an orthogonal Varimax rotation on the intercorrelation matrices. All principle component analyses revealed an identical two-factor structure for each clock condition when analyzed separately. All clock scores, therefore, were summed to obtain a grand total clock score for each subject. These grand total clock scores and neuropsychological test scores were then re-analyzed by the principal components analysis followed by an orthogonal Varimax rotation. The unrotated and rotated factor loadings are presented in Table 2-6. Two factors accounted for 53.4 percent of the variance in the data. Test scores from the WAIS-R subtests, Information, Block Design, Picture Completion, and Arithmetic, as well as total scores from the Controlled Oral Word Association test, loaded on Factor 1 (Table 2-6). The total score of the clock-drawing conditions loaded on Factor 2, along with the score for the copy condition of the Rey-Osterrieth Complex Figure, WAIS-R Block Design subtest score, and the number of perseverative responses from the Wisconsin Card Sorting Test (WCST).

To determine the effect of cognitive impairment on clock drawing, groups of elderly subjects with and without dementia were administered the examiner's clocks. The presence or absence of dementia was defined by the subject's score on the Mattis Dementia Rating Scale (DRS) (Mattis, 1988). As suggested by Montgomery and Costa (1983) a score of less than 123 was considered as indicating dementia. Group composition was as follows: Group 1 consisted of 18 nondemented, elderly subjects living in a senior citizen's residence. Group 2 consisted of 20 subjects with Parkinson's disease but without dementia. Group 3 consisted of 14 subjects with Parkinson's disease with dementia. Group 4 was comprised of 13 subjects with Alzheimer's disease whose DRS score fell below 123.

Table 2-4. Percentage of Subjects with a Given Total Clock Score

6:45 Free-Drawn Clock

Age Group

Score	20–29 %	20–29 Cum.%	30–39 %	30–39 Cum.%	40–49 %	40–49 Cum.%	50–59 %	50–59 Cum.%	60–69 %	60–69 Cum.%	70–79 %	70–79 Cum.%	80–90 %	80–90 Cum.%
0														
1														
2														
3														
4														
5														
6											1.9	1.9		
7													2.4	2.4
8													2.4	4.9
9											1.9	3.7	4.9	9.8
10											5.6	9.3	2.4	12.2
11							1.9	1.9			1.9	11.1	2.4	14.6
12									5.3	5.3	5.6	16.7	9.8	24.4
13	7.5	7.5	2.5	2.5			9.6	11.5	12.0	17.3	9.3	25.9	7.3	31.7
14	15.0	22.5	20.0	22.5	23.1	23.1	23.1	34.6	32.0	49.3	33.3	59.3	34.1	65.9
15	77.5	100.0	77.5	100.0	76.9	100.0	65.4	100.0	50.7	100.0	40.7	100.0	34.1	100.0

Table 2-4. (Continued)

6:05 Pre-Drawn Clock

Score	Age Group													
	20–29		30–39		40–49		50–59		60–69		70–79		80–90	
	%	Cum.%	%	Cum.%	%	Cum.%	%	Cum.%	%	Cum.%	%	Cum.%	%	Cum.%
0														
1														
2														
3														
4														
5														
6													4.9	4.9
7											1.7	1.7		
8											5.1	6.8	7.3	12.2
9											6.8	13.6	4.9	17.1
10					2.6	2.6	1.9	1.9	1.3	1.3	8.5	22.1	12.2	29.3
11	2.5	2.5	5.0	5.0	5.1	7.7	7.7	9.6	15.8	17.1	16.9	39.0	9.8	39.1
12	22.5	25.0	20.0	25.0	17.9	25.6	25.0	34.6	26.3	43.4	32.2	71.2	31.7	70.7
13	75.0	100.0	75.0	100.0	74.4	100.0	65.4	100.0	56.6	100.0	28.8	100.0	29.3	100.0

(continued)

Table 2-4. *(Continued)*

11:10 Examiner Clock

Score	Age Group													
	20–29		30–39		40–49		50–59		60–69		70–79		80–90	
	%	Cum.%	%	Cum.%	%	Cum.%	%	Cum.%	%	Cum.%	%	Cum.%	%	Cum.%
0														
1														
2			2.5	2.5							1.7	1.7	2.4	2.4
3											3.4	5.1	4.9	7.3
4											1.7	6.8	2.4	9.8
5									1.3	1.3	1.7	8.5	2.4	12.2
6			2.5	5.0							1.7	10.2		
7											5.1	15.3		
8							1.9	1.9	1.3	2.6	1.7	16.9	2.4	14.6
9			5.0	10.0	7.5	7.5	5.8	7.7	3.9	6.6	10.2	27.1	12.2	26.8
10	20.0	20.0	15.0	25.0	17.5	25.0	23.1	30.8	27.6	34.2	27.1	54.2	41.5	68.3
11	80.0	100.0	75.0	100.0	75.0	100.0	69.2	100.0	65.8	100.0	45.8	100.0	31.7	100.0

8:20 Examiner Clock

	Age Group												
	20–29		30–39		40–49		50–59		60–69		70–79		80–90	
Score	%	Cum.%	%	Cum.%	%	Cum.%	%	Cum.%	%	Cum.%	%	Cum.%	%	Cum.%
0														
1														
2													2.4	2.4
3			2.5	2.5	2.5	2.5					1.7	1.7	2.4	4.9
4											3.4	5.1		
5											3.4	8.5	2.4	7.3
6													4.9	12.2
7											5.1	13.6		
8	5.0	5.0	2.5	5.0					1.3	1.3	5.1	18.6		
9	5.0	10.0	5.0	10.0			5.8	5.8	6.6	7.9	5.1	23.7		
10	15.0	25.0	15.0	25.0	27.5	30.0	17.3	23.1	31.6	39.5	22.0	45.8	29.3	51.2
11	75.0	100.0	75.0	100.0	70.0	100.0	76.9	100.0	60.5	100.0	54.2	100.0	48.8	100.0

(continued)

Table 2-4. (Continued)

3:00 Examiner Clock

Age Group

Score	20–29		30–39		40–49		50–59		60–69		70–79		80–90	
	%	Cum.%	%	Cum.%	%	Cum.%	%	Cum.%	%	Cum.%	%	Cum.%	%	Cum.%
0														
1														
2														
3											3.4	3.4	4.9	4.9
4														
5											5.1	8.5	2.4	7.3
6													2.4	9.8
7											3.4	11.9	2.4	12.2
8											1.7	13.6		
9			2.5	2.5	5.0	5.0	3.8	3.8	7.9	7.9	5.1	18.6	9.8	22.0
10	17.5	17.5	35.0	37.5	22.5	27.5	19.2	23.1	23.7	31.6	33.9	52.5	31.7	53.7
11	82.5	100.0	62.5	100.0	72.5	100.0	76.9	100.0	68.4	100.0	47.5	100.0	46.3	100.0

TABLE 2-5. Intercorrelation of Tasks Corrected for Age

| | Free-drawn | Pre-drawn | Examiner 11:10 | Examiner 8:20 | Examiner 3:00 | WAIS-R | | | | |
						Info	Arith	BD	PC	Full
Free-drawn										
Pre-drawn	.50									
Examiner 11:10	.32	.22								
Examiner 8:20	.33	.20	.40							
Examiner 3:00	.20	.21	.22	.48						
WAIS-R										
Info	.26	.26	.13	.28	.24					
Arith	.18	.17	.14	.17	.11	.35				
BD	.31	.26	.21	.37	.27	.47	.31			
PC	.21	.27	.07	.24	.30	.45	.27	.51		
Full	.31	.31	.20	.38	.31	.75	.62	.77	.75	
Wisconsin Card Sorting Test										
No. Categories	.10	.14	.08	.16	.14	.22	.24	.43	.28	.40
Correct	.14	.10	.12	.08	.03	-.08	.03	.05	.00	.02
Error	-.16	-.12	-.09	-.18	-.17	-.28	-.33	-.44	-.32	-.46
Pers resp	-.18	-.13	-.08	-.19	-.18	-.27	-.33	-.41	-.32	-.45
Pers error	-.17	-.14	-.09	-.19	-.18	-.29	-.33	-.42	-.33	-.47
Nonpers error	-.08	-.05	-.03	-.12	-.14	-.28	-.28	-.40	-.26	-.41
No. Cards sorted	-.12	-.11	-.06	-.14	-.15	-.30	-.29	-.43	-.33	-.46
Rey-Osterrieth Complex Figure										
Copy	.27	.18	.23	.33	.26	.23	.22	.34	.31	.38
Immed	.37	.25	.22	.34	.27	.44	.29	.48	.43	.56
Delay	.30	.25	.23	.30	.23	.47	.30	.48	.41	.56
FAS	.20	.14	.05	.20	.12	.34	.33	.28	.25	.40

(continued)

TABLE 2-5. Intercorrelation of Tasks Corrected for Age (*Continued*)

| | Wisconsin Card Sort | | | | | | | Rey-Osterrieth Complex Figure | | | |
	Sorts	Correct	Error	Pers resp	Pers error	Nonpers error	Cards	Copy	Imm	Delay	FAS
Free-drawn											
Pre-drawn											
Examiner 11:10											
Examiner 8:20											
Examiner 3:00											
WAIS-R											
Info											
Arith											
BD											
PC											
Full											
Wisconsin Card Sorting Test											
No. Categories											
Correct	.18										
Error	−.85	−.03									
Pers resp	−.78	.00	.92								
Pers error	−.79	.01	.93	.99							
Nonpers error	−.78	.11	.89	.71	.72						
No. Cards sorted	−.80	.28	.91	.86	.88	.87					
Rey-Osterrieth Complex Figure											
Copy	.24	.12	−.30	−.31	−.31	−.23	−.24				
Immed	.25	.01	−.30	−.36	−.36	−.22	−.31	.36			
Delay	.26	.01	−.30	−.36	−.36	−.21	−.30	.35	.88		
FAS	.10	−.02	−.15	−.17	−.18	−.09	−.12	.14	.23	.25	

Table 2-6.   Principal Component Analysis: Clock Drawing and Neuropsychological Tests

	Factor	
Unrotated Factor Pattern	**1**	**2**
Total Clock Score	.51	−.55
Rey-Osterrieth Copy	.58	−.52
WCST Perseverative Responses	−.57	.30
WAIS-R Block Design	.76	.01
WAIS-R Information	.71	.32
WAIS-R Arithmetic	.61	.26
WAIS-R Picture Completion	.71	.14
FAS Total	.52	.50
Eigenvalue	3.16	1.11

	Factor		
Rotated Factor Pattern	**1**	**2**	**Communality**
Total Clock Store	.05	.75	.57
Rey-Osterrieth Copy	.13	.77	.61
WCST Perservative Response	−.26	−.59	.42
WAIS-R Block Design	.60	.46	.57
WAIS-R Information	.76	.19	.61
WAIS-R Arithmetic	.64	.18	.44
WAIS-R Picture Completion	.65	.33	.53
FAS Total	.72	−.07	.52
Variance explained by each factor	2.36	1.91	

Factor loading required for significance > .43
Total variance accounted for by 2 factors = 53.4%

Between-group differences were analyzed by an ANCOVA using age as a covariate. Results are summarized in Table 2-7. There was a significant group effect for all mean total clock scores for each clock condition. Subsequent pairwise comparisons revealed that the mean total clock scores for the normal controls and nondemented Parkinson's patients did not differ significantly. Both the demented Parkinson's patients and Alzheimer's patients obtained significantly lower mean total clock scores relative to the normal control group, however.

To evaluate the ability of the clock drawings to discriminate demented from nondemented subjects, a stepwise logistic regression was performed on the data obtained from the groups of subjects described above. Total clock scores for all three examiner's clocks were summed to obtain a grand total score, with a maximum possible of 33. Optimal discrimination was found using a cutoff score of less than 28 (chi-square = 28.31; $df = 1$). The sensitivity of the cutoff of less than 28 points was .85 and the specificity was .82; only 15 percent of the demented subjects obtained clock scores

Table 2-7.   Total Clock Score.

	Examiner Clock Condition				
	11:10	**8:20**	**3:00**	**N**	
Nondemented controls	9.5 ± 1.9	9.6 ± 2.3	9.9 ± 1.4	18	—
Parkinson's disease without dementia	9.4 ± 2.6	9.4 ± 2.3	9.9 ± 1.8	20	NS
Parkinson's disease with dementia	4.5 ± 2.9	4.9 ± 3.3	5.8 ± 3.8	14	$p < .05$
Alzheimer's disease	5.2 ± 3.6	5.2 ± 3.4	5.8 ± 3.6	13	$p < .05$

above the cutoff and only 18 percent of the nondemented subjects obtained scores below the cutoff. Lowering the cutoff scores resulted in a much lower gain in specificity at the cost of a marked decrease in sensitivity.

We also administered the free-drawn condition to the same groups of well elderly, nondemented patients with Parkinson's disease, and demented Parkinson's and Alzheimer's patients described above to evaluate the discriminability of our scoring system. A stepwise logistic regression was also performed on the free-drawn clock data. Optimal discrimination was found using a cutoff of 12 out of a possible 15 total points (chi-square = 23.38; $df = 1$). The cutoff of less than 12 gave a sensitivity of .78 and a specificity of .82. Although the sensitivity was somewhat lower than that obtained for the examiner's clock condition, overall the discrimination was equivalent.

Discussion

Our first goals were to acquire normative data on clock drawing at different ages and to develop a clinically useful scoring system. The descriptors that were initially developed were comprehensive but unwieldy for practical purposes. A smaller subset of the original descriptors was selected, which represented critical attributes of clocks and responses that were highly likely to occur in the normative sample. This set of "critical items" allowed us to develop an objective scoring system for the conditions of the free-drawn, pre-drawn, and examiner clocks. Interrater reliability of the scoring system tended to be very high. Scores tended to remain stable across two separate testing conditions although for the pre-drawn clock condition the scores tended to be higher on the second test.

Age had a significant effect on clock-drawing ability, with the greatest decrease in scores occurring above the age of 70. The most common errors included incorrect representation of the proportion of the hands and incorrect placement of the minute hand. This makes intuitive sense because hand length and minute number are the most abstract features of a clock.

The results of the principal component analysis revealed that all clock-drawing tests loaded heavily on a single factor along with scores from the copy condition of the Rey-Osterrieth Complex Figure, WAIS-R Block Design, and perseverative responses of the

Wisconsin Card Sorting Test. Furthermore, intercorrelations among clock drawings and the other supposed measures of visuoconstructional or visuoperceptual abilities, such as the Rey-Osterrieth copy score and WAIS-R Block Design, were statistically significant. These relationships suggest that clock drawing is a test of visual-analytic ability. More specifically, it evaluates the collective processes required to retrieve the representation of time from memory and translate it into a familiar visuospatial relationship.

Performance on the clock-drawing test is negatively affected by the presence of generalized cognitive impairment and can be used to discriminate groups of cognitively impaired from nonimpaired subjects. Using the scoring system based upon the critical items from the normative study, we were able to define an optimal cutoff score based on the total scores of the three examiner clock conditions that was both sensitive and specific to the presence of dementia. A total score of less than 28 correctly identified 85 percent of demented subjects and misidentified only 18 percent of nondemented subjects. For the free-drawn clock condition we found that a cutoff of less than 12 points identified 78 percent of demented patients and misidentified only 18 percent of nondemented subjects.

Our results are consistent with those reported by other investigators, although we did not attempt a direct comparison between our scoring system and others that have been published. Nussbaum, Fields, & Starratt (1992) compared the scoring systems of Rouleau et al. (1992), Wolf-Klein et al. (1989), and Sunderland et al. (1989) and found significant and high intertest correlations that varied from .74 to .92. Upon reviewing the various studies it appears that the most reliable scoring systems are those that have utilized an ordinal scale such as ours. All scoring systems place emphasis and weighting on the ability to set time correctly. Our own system assigns the most points to the features relating to the hands—e.g., number of hands, relative length, placement, and joining. Thereby, the ability to reproduce these features is given the greatest weight. This is particularly true of our examiner clock condition where only the elements relating to the hands are scored. Taking only these elements into consideration, we found very good sensitivity and specificity.

To obtain a complete measure of the abilities involved in clock drawing, we recommend that all conditions used in the present study be given. This includes the "6:45" free-drawn clock, as well as the "6:05" pre-drawn clock and the "11:10," "8:20," and "3:00" examiner clocks. The total time to complete all three conditions is approximately 6 to 10 minutes. Moreover, scoring is relatively reliable and quick.

One aspect of clock drawing that was not dealt with in the normative study relates to the value of specific types of errors on clock drawing for identifying or discriminating specific neurological dysfunction. This question can only be addressed by studying clock drawing in patients with cognitive dysfunction due to neurological disorders such as Alzheimer's and Parkinson's disease, as well as patients with circumscribed focal brain lesions. This will be the subject of the following chapters. The normative study, however, will serve as an important basis of comparison for evaluating the clocks drawn by the cognitively impaired subjects.

3. Dementia and Related Disorders

Although clock drawing is a relatively simple task to administer, the multifactorial cognitive mechanisms underlying clock drawing make this task very sensitive to the widespread disruption of brain systems that are affected by the various forms of dementia. Moreover, clock drawing is a reliable measure of cognitive dysfunction, as demonstrated by Shulman, Sheldetsky, & Silver, 1986; Sunderland et al., 1989; Nussbaum et al., 1992; and Tuokko et al., 1992. As a result, clock drawing is being increasingly used in the assessment of dementia by physicians, neuropsychologists, occupational therapists, and other health care workers involved in the evaluation of patients with cognitive deficits (Dastoor, Schwartz, & Kurzman, 1991; Henderson et al., 1989; Huntzinger et al., 1992; Kirk & Kertesz, 1991; Mendez, Ala, & Underwood, 1992; Shulman et al., 1986; Sunderland et al., 1989; Wolf-Klein et al., 1989).

Whereas our normative study defines the spectrum of clocks that normal subjects draw at different ages, it does not encompass the errors produced by cognitively impaired patients with dementia. Although the literature on clock drawing in patients with dementia is extremely limited, there is some information about performance on this task in Alzheimer's disease (Albert & Moss, 1984; Rouleau et al., 1992; Sunderland et al., 1989; Tuokko et al., 1992; Wolf-Klein et al., 1989), multi-infarct dementia (Wolf-Klein et al., 1989), and Huntington's disease (Rouleau et al., 1992).

Wolf-Klein and colleagues studied a large group of subjects with Alzheimer's disease, as well as a smaller group of subjects with multi-infarct dementia and Alzheimer's disease combined with multi-infarct dementia. Subjects had a mean age of 76.8 years with a range from 58–99 years. They were presented with a pre-drawn circle that was 4 inches in diameter and asked to draw a clock. The abnormalities in Alzheimer's disease included irrelevant figures such as words, irrelevant spatial arrangement of the numbers, counterclockwise rotation, absence of numbers, and perseveration. In contrast, subjects with multi-infarct dementia performed better than those with Alzheimer's disease. Abnormalities in the multi-infarct dementia group consisted primarily of errors in the numbers, as well as impaired spacing of the numbers. The Mini-Mental State Examination score was higher, however, in patients with multi-infarct dementia as compared to Alzheimer's disease (19.4 ± 7.4 vs. 12.8 ± 8.1).

Rouleau et al. (1992) studied clock-drawing ability in patients with Alzheimer's disease and Huntington's disease. Both groups had been equated for severity of dementia on the Mattis Dementia Rating Scale (DRS). The scores were 114.68 ± 20.07 and 110.08 ± 27.09 for the Alzheimer and Huntington subjects, respectively. Subjects with Alzheimer's disease had a mean age of 71 ± 6.7 years, whereas subjects with Huntington's disease had a mean age of 49.84 ± 12.70 years. Administration of the clock-drawing test included both a command and copy condition. In the command condition, subjects were presented with an 8½-by-11-inch blank sheet of paper and given the following instructions: "I would like you to draw a clock, put in all the numbers, and set the hands for 10 after 11." In the copy condition, subjects were presented with a 3-inch diameter clock that contained all the numbers and that had the time set at "10 after 11." The scoring system consisted of a 10-point quantitative scale and a 6-item qualitative scale. The quantitative scale was comprised of measurements for the integrity of the clock face, presence and sequencing of the numbers, and the presence and placement of the hands. The qualitative error analysis focused on the size of the clock, graphic difficulties, stimulus-bound responses, conceptual deficits, spatial and/or planning deficits, and perseveration.

Rouleau and colleagues found that patients with Alzheimer's disease and Huntington's disease were significantly impaired compared to normal controls based upon an overall quantitative score for the command and copy condition. Subjects with Alzheimer's disease, however, performed better to copy than to command, whereas those with Huntington's disease were equally impaired on both conditions. Albert and Moss (1984) also noted that patients with Alzheimer's disease performed better on clock drawing to copy than to command. In contrast to the quantitative scores, the qualitative error analysis showed different profiles for each of the groups. Patients with Alzheimer's disease tended to draw larger clocks to command, showed conceptual deficits, tended to write numbers outside the clocks, and had more perseverative and stimulus-bound responses. Patients with Huntington's disease tended to draw smaller clocks to command, showed moderate to severe graphic deficits, and had planning deficits in the spatial layout of the numbers.

Sunderland et al. (1989) also found that clock drawing was significantly impaired in Alzheimer's disease compared to normals. These researchers asked subjects to "First, draw a clock with all the numbers on it. Second, put the hands on the clock to make it read 2:45." They rated the clocks on a 10-point scale with "10" representing the best clock and "1" representing the worst response. A score of 6 to 10 indicated that the clock face and numbers were generally intact but that there were errors in hand placement. A score of 1 to 5 applied to clocks in which the face and numbers were not intact. They found that the majority of subjects with Alzheimer's disease drew abnormal clocks that were rated with a score of less than 6 with a clock face and numbers that were not intact. No subject with Alzheimer's disease was able to draw a perfect clock. They also found significant correlations between the mean clock score in Alzheimer's disease and measures of dementia severity. As noted by Rouleau and colleagues (1992), however, the scoring system adopted by Sunderland and colleagues assumes that the ability to draw hands on a clock is affected first and that difficulty representing numbers and the clock face occur later. This assumption is not always correct.

Tuokko et al. (1992) compared clock drawing in patients with Alzheimer's disease to age- and gender-matched normal subjects. They assessed performance under each of three conditions comprised of clock drawing, clock setting, and clock reading. For clock drawing, they asked subjects to put the numbers on a pre-drawn circle and to set the time at "10 past 11." For clock setting, the subjects were required to set the hands at various different times on a pre-drawn clock face that had no numbers but did contain marks at the number locations. For clock reading, subjects were required to tell the time on a clock containing marks at the sites of the number locations and hands.

The scoring system used by Tuokko and colleagues consisted of seven error categories for clock drawing: These were omissions, perseverations, rotations, misplacements, distortions, substitutions, and additions. The types of errors within each category were defined. For example, perseveration included repetition of numbers, hand perseverations, and sequence of number perseverations. The scoring system for clock setting consisted of one point for placing each hand correctly and one point for the correct proportion of the hands. Clock reading was scored by awarding points on the basis of the numbers of hands read correctly. Tuokko and co-workers found that the subjects with Alzheimer's disease were significantly impaired on clock drawing, clock setting, and clock reading. Analysis of the error types on clock drawing showed that patients with Alzheimer's disease made significantly more errors of omission and misplacements of numbers compared to normals.

Henderson, Mack, and Williams (1989) used clock drawing as one of their measures of visuoconstructive function in a study designed to identify predictors of spatial disorientation—i.e., a tendency to wander and get lost—in Alzheimer's disease. They studied two groups of patients with Alzheimer's disease, 11 with spatial disorientation and 17 without. The groups did not differ from each other with regard to age, education, sex, duration of symptoms, or severity of the dementia (Mini-Mental State Examination). Nor did they differ on such neuropsychological measures as digit span (WAIS-R) and naming (Boston Naming Test). Henderson and colleagues did find, however, that drawing and memory tasks could differentiate between the two groups of Alzheimer's patients. The drawing tasks were the clock and house drawing to verbal command and to copy conditions from the Spatial Quantitative Battery of the Boston Diagnostic Aphasia Examination.

Henderson and colleagues created a simplified scoring system yielding a maximum score of 5 points for each "10 after 11" clock drawn (one point each for presence of an outer contour, relatively circular face, symmetrical number placement, correct numbers, and correct time). Scoring for the house drawing was similar, one point each for outer form, presence of a roof, two sides, and accuracy of perspective, yielding a maximum of 4 points for each house drawn. The total drawing score, along with the delayed recall of a given address from the Blessed Information-Memory-Concentration Test, proved the best predictors of spatial disorientation, accounting for 41 percent of the variance. The authors then argued that, because spatial disorientation—i.e., wandering, or getting lost—is a behavior not commonly seen in association with either unilateral focal posterior lesions in the right hemisphere or with memory problems alone, only a combination of visuoconstructive problems and delayed recall can account for spatial disorientation.

It remains to be seen whether clock drawing alone, but with a scoring system comparable to ours, and some memory tasks that differentiate between encoding and retrieval, can more effectively differentiate between patients with anterior versus posterior lesions in the right hemisphere. This kind of differentiation would bring us closer to understanding the underlying mechanism in spatially disoriented behavior and would have implications for more effective patient management.

In our own series of patients, we applied the scoring system developed in the normative study in a systematic evaluation of patients with Alzheimer's disease and Parkinson's disease with dementia. The clocks were compared to those drawn by normal controls and by patients with Parkinson's disease without dementia. Patients with Alzheimer's disease all met criteria for probable Alzheimer's disease established by the National Institute of Neurological and Communicative Disorders and Stroke and the Alzheimer's Disease and Related Disorders Association (NINCDS-ADRDA) (McKhann, Drachman, Folstein et al., 1984). The Parkinson's patients also met standard diagnostic criteria (Adams & Victor, 1989; Weiner & Lang, 1989). General level of cognitive function was assessed using the Mattis Dementia Rating Scale (DRS) (Coblentz et al., 1973; Mattis, 1988). The DRS correlates well with the Weschler Adult Intelligence Scale and measures cognitive function along the factors of attention, perseveration, constructional ability, conceptualization, and memory. Because a score of less than 123 has been used as a cutoff for dementia (Montgomery & Costa, 1983), we applied this criterion to separate the patients with Parkinson's disease into subgroups with dementia and without dementia. All of the subjects with Alzheimer's disease had a DRS of less than 123. The age and education of the subjects are shown in Table 3-1. The normal controls were selected from the normative study and were comprised of all subjects over 60 years of age.

Clock-drawing ability was assessed using the same procedures as in the normative study. These consisted of a free-drawn and pre-drawn condition, as well as three examiner conditions.

1. *Free-drawn clock condition.* Subjects were presented with a blank sheet of

Table 3-1. Age and Education of Subject Groups

Groups	Age	Years of Education
Alzheimer's disease (n=13)		
Mean (range)	72.9 (63–80)	11.7 (8–16)
SD	5.6	2.4
Parkinson's disease with dementia (n=14)		
Mean (range)	77.4 (74–82)	7.8 (0–17)
SD	2.9	5.7
Parkinson's disease without dementia (n=20)		
Mean (range)	68.8 (61–78)	14.6 (7–21)
SD	5.0	4.0
Normal controls (n=176)		
Mean (range)	72.0 (60–90)	13.6 (0–23)
SD	7.7	3.6

8¹/₂-by-11-inch white paper and given the following instructions: "I would like you to draw a clock and put in all the numbers." After the subject had done this, the examiner said, "Now I would like you to set the time at quarter to 7." After completing the free-drawn clock, all subjects were asked to complete the pre-drawn clock.

2. *Pre-drawn clock condition.* Subjects were given a sheet of paper with a pre-drawn circle measuring 11 cm (4¹/₄ in) in diameter and instructed to "Put the numbers on the clock and set the time at 5 after 6." Next, the three examiner clocks were administered.

3. *Examiner clock conditions.* For each of the three conditions, subjects were presented with a sheet of 8¹/₂-by-11-inch white paper with a pre-drawn clock face with the numbers already on it. The diameter of the clock face was 11 cm. The height of the numbers was 6 mm (¹/₄ in). The examiner instructed the subjects to set the time at "10 after 11," "20 after 8," or "3 o'clock" in a counterbalanced order on each of the examiner-drawn clocks.

Total Clock Scores

The free-drawn, pre-drawn, and three examiner clocks produced by the different subject groups were compared on the critical items outlined in the normative chapter (see Table 2-2). For the free-drawn clocks, a total score was calculated using the critical items for clock contour, numbers, hands, and center (maximum score = 15). The total score for the pre-drawn clocks was based upon the critical items for numbers, hands, and center (maximum score = 13). For the examiner clocks, it was based upon the critical items for hands and center (maximum score = 11).

Table 3-2 shows the mean total clock scores obtained by the subject groups on the free-drawn, pre-drawn, and examiner clock conditions, as well as the results of a statistical comparison between the subject groups on the different clock conditions. As shown in Table 3-2, subjects with Alzheimer's disease and Parkinson's disease with dementia were significantly impaired on all of the clock conditions.

Performance on Different Clock Conditions

The free-drawn, pre-drawn, and three examiner clock conditions were analyzed using the critical items developed in the normative study. Comparisons for each critical item were made among each of the groups with Alzheimer's disease, Parkinson's disease with dementia, and Parkinson's disease without dementia, respectively, and the normal controls using the Wilcoxon test, a nonparametric procedure.

FREE-DRAWN CLOCKS (6:45)

Table 3-3 shows the performance profiles of the subjects with Alzheimer's disease, Parkinson's disease with dementia, and Parkinson's disease without dementia, as well as the normal controls, on each of the critical items developed in the normative study for contour, numbers, hands, and center. Although the free-drawn clock is the only

Table 3-2. Total Clock Scores

	AD (n=13)	DPD (n=14)	NDPD (n=20)	Normals (n=176)[†]
Free-Drawn Clock (max=15)				
Mean	8.3*	8.1*	13.4	13.9
SD	3.8	3.4	2.4	1.6
Pre-Drawn Clock (max=13)				
Mean	6.8*	7.1*	11.1	11.8
SD	3.9	2.7	3.2	1.5
Examiner Clock (max=11)				
11:10				
Mean	5.2*	4.5*	9.5	9.9
SD	3.7	2.9	2.6	1.9
8:20				
Mean	5.2*	4.9*	9.4	10.1
SD	3.6	3.3	2.3	1.8
3:00				
Mean	5.8*	5.8*	9.9	10.1
SD	3.6	3.9	1.8	1.6

AD, Alzheimer's disease.

DPD, Parkinson's disease with dementia.

NDPD, Parkinson's disease without dementia.

[†] n=170 for free-drawn condition.

* p < 0.0001 for AD and DPD vs. NDPD and normal controls, respectively. (Comparisons were based upon a separate ANCOVA for each clock condition with age as a covariate. Subsequent between-group comparisons were carried out using the Least Squares Means Procedure).

condition that provides information about contour, it should be stressed that drawing the numbers may be confounded by a poor contour. Similarly, drawing the hands and center may be affected by both a poor contour and impaired drawing of the numbers.

Contour Whereas all patients with Alzheimer's disease who had a DRS above 70 were generally able to draw an acceptable contour, this was not the case for the subjects with Parkinson's disease with dementia who had comparable scores on the DRS. In contrast, the range of contour sizes drawn by patients with Parkinson's disease with dementia was similar to those drawn by patients with Alzheimer's disease. Contours ranged in size from being too small to contain the numbers to being quite large (Figure 3-1A–D). Although the more severely impaired subjects tended to draw smaller contours, this was not a consistent finding.

Subjects with Alzheimer's disease tended to draw clock contours that were generally circular in shape. Contours drawn by patients with Parkinson's dementia, however, tended to be less symmetrical and more oval than those drawn by Alzheimer's patients (Figure 3-2A,B). This likely reflects the motor deficits characteristic of Parkinson's disease.

Parkinson's disease with dementia is associated with prominent frontal system deficits that have been well documented using standardized and experimental neuropsycho-

TABLE 3-3.   Free-Drawn Clocks

	Percentage of Subjects with a Given Response[†]			
	AD (n=13)	DPD (n=14)	NDPD (n=20)	Normals (n=170)
Contour				
Acceptable	100.0	85.7**	100.0	100.0
Not too small, overdrawn or reproduced repeatedly	76.9**	91.7*	100.0 (n=12)	98.2
Numbers				
Only numbers 1–12 present	53.8**	50.0*	95.0	95.3
Only Arabic numbers used	83.3** (n=12)	92.3*	85.0* (n=13)	95.9
Numbers in correct order	75.0** (n=12)	84.6* (n=13)	100.0	100.0
Numbers drawn without rotating paper	100.0 (n=12)	100.0 (n=13)	100.0	94.7
Numbers in correct position	33.3** (n=12)	23.1* (n=13)	80.0	79.4
Numbers all inside contour	83.3 (n=12)	61.5** (n=13)	80.0	92.9
Hands				
Two hands present	30.8**	35.7**	85.0	94.7
Hour target number indicated	69.2**	57.1**	95.0	95.9
Minute target number indicated	23.1**	14.3**	85.0	89.4
Hands in correct proportion	0.0* (n=4)	60.0 (n=5)	70.6 (n=17)	76.6 (n=158)
No superfluous markings	46.2**	64.3	90.0	88.8
Hands relatively joined	100.0 (n=4)	80.0 (n=5)	100.0 (n=17)	98.8 (n=161)
Center				
Center is present (drawn or inferred)	46.2**	28.6**	100.0	95.9

[†] Percentage based only on subjects in whom the item could be scored. The sample size is shown in parentheses when less than original total.

$* p \leq 0.01.$

$** p \leq 0.001.$

logical measures (Bowen, Kamienny, Burns, & Yahr, 1975; Cools et al., 1984; Flowers, 1982; Flowers & Robertson, 1985; Freedman & Oscar-Berman, 1986; Lees & Smith, 1983; Taylor, Saint-Cyr, & Lang, 1986). Figure 3-2C provides an example of frontal system deficits in a patient with Parkinson's disease and dementia that were demonstrated on clock drawing. This patient did not draw a contour but drew a hand that looked like a "mouth" on the "face" of the clock.

Subjects with Parkinson's disease without dementia were able to draw acceptable contours that were large enough to contain the numbers, were not overdrawn, and were not reproduced repeatedly. Although some of the contours were quite small, these

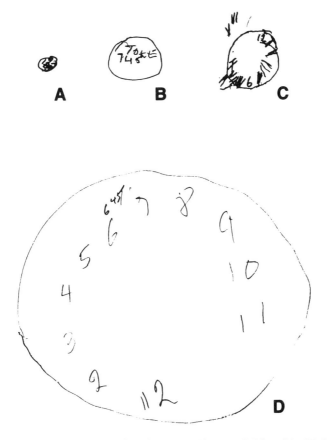

A   B   C

D

Figure 3–1 (A) Alzheimer's disease, female, age = 79 years, DRS = 91. (B) Parkinson's disease with dementia, male, age = 75 years, DRS = 67. (C) Parkinson's disease with dementia, male, age = 77 years, DRS = 97. (D) Alzheimer's disease, male, age = 78 years, DRS = 106.

subjects were able to compensate by writing appropriately small numbers that fit into the circle. Parkinson's patients without dementia, however, drew the same types of asymmetrical and oval contours seen in the Parkinson's patients with dementia. Again, this can be attributed to the motor deficits in this group.

Numbers The most common errors in the patients with Alzheimer's disease and Parkinson's disease with dementia consisted of omitting numbers, adding extra numbers, ordering numbers incorrectly, and positioning the numbers poorly (Figure 3-2A,B). As expected, these errors were most common in the more severely impaired subjects. In addition, patients with Parkinson's disease and dementia frequently placed numbers outside the clock contour (Figure 3-3A).

Subjects who omitted numbers often did so because the contour was too small to contain them all. Numbers may, however, still be omitted even when there is sufficient

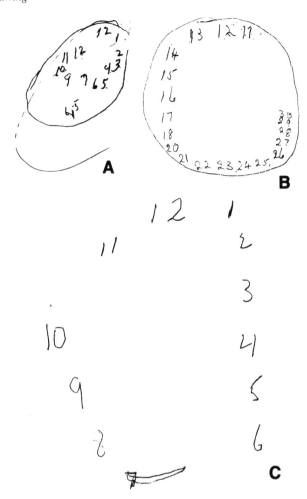

Figure 3–2   (A) Parkinson's disease with dementia, male, age = 81 years, DRS = 100.
(B) Alzheimer's disease, female, age = 73 years, DRS = 86. (C) Parkinson's disease with
dementia, male, age = 74 years, DRS = 106.

room on the clock face (Figure 3-3A,B). Subjects added extra numbers for a variety of
reasons including inattention to a previously written number (Figure 3-2A) and perseveration on writing a number sequence (Figure 3-2B). Patients who omitted numbers,
added extra numbers, or placed them in the wrong order tended to have more severe
dementia.

Although most patients with dementia drew only Arabic numerals, a small percentage drew Roman numerals combined with Arabic numerals (Figure 3-1C). Whereas
normal subjects draw Roman numeral clocks on rare occasions (only one subject in
normative study), they never combine Roman and Arabic numbers on the same clock.

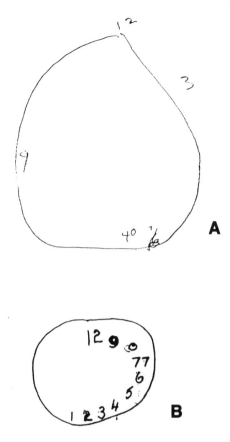

Figure 3–3   (A) Parkinson's disease with dementia, female, age = 79 years. DRS = 121.
(B) Alzheimer's disease, female, age = 63 years, DRS = 103.

They may, however, combine Arabic numerals and strokes at the sites of the numbers. Patients with dementia may do this as well. For some, the strokes are placed first to indicate where the numbers should appear.

Placement of numbers in the correct position was the critical item for numbers on which normals had the greatest difficulty. Not surprisingly, it was also the critical item for numbers on which patients with dementia also did the most poorly. In contrast to normals, however, many subjects with dementia who positioned their numbers poorly also tended either to add or omit numbers.

It is of interest that rotation of the paper while placing numbers was not characteristic of patients with either Alzheimer's or Parkinson's disease with dementia on the free-drawn clocks. Instead, rotation of the paper appeared to be related more to aging and was seen in approximately 10 percent of normals over the age of 70 (see normative study, Chapter 2).

In contrast to the subjects with dementia, the Parkinson's patients without dementia drew numbers very well. In some cases they tended to draw a combination of Arabic numbers and strokes. This is not a pathological response, however. There was also a tendency for Parkinson's patients without dementia who had DRS scores in the lower range of normal to place some numbers outside and some inside the clock contour. As indicated above, drawing numbers outside the clock contour was a significant occurrence in patients with Parkinson's disease who have dementia. Thus, when patients with Parkinson's disease without dementia begin to place one or more numbers outside the contour, the question of a deterioration in cognitive function should be raised.

Hands   The majority of patients with Alzheimer's disease and Parkinson's disease with dementia failed to draw two hands on the clock face. As expected, it was the less severely affected subjects who were able to draw both hands. The deficit underlying the ability to draw hands is most likely due to conceptual difficulties rather than memory loss since the subjects were instructed to set the time after they had drawn their clocks.

In patients with Alzheimer's disease, there was a clear relation between a preserved ability to draw two hands and the ability to draw an acceptable contour and to place all the numbers accurately on the clock. In the demented Parkinson's patients who drew two hands, however, the contours were not as good as those drawn by patients with Alzheimer's disease. Also, the numbers tended not to be as well drawn.

In both dementia groups, more subjects were able to indicate the hour target number as compared to the minute target number because indication of the hour target number does not require recoding from one number to another. In contrast, for a "quarter to 7" the "quarter" must be recoded as a "9." Those subjects who did indicate the hour number, either by a hand or a mark, tended to target the correct number regardless of whether it was in the correct position on the clock face. Subjects who were too impaired to indicate the hour target number were generally not able to give any indication of the time at all.

Because indicating the minute target number requires recoding from "one quarter" to a "9," this aspect of the clock-drawing task is very sensitive to frontal system deficits. This is well illustrated in Figure 3-4A in which the "one quarter" is written beside the "4" in a concrete fashion. Other examples of frontal responses seen in the more severely impaired subjects include writing "745" across the clock face without drawing any hands (Figure 3-1B), or writing "645" between the numerals "6" and "7" (Figure 3-1D).

Superfluous markings are defined as any markings not necessary for the indication of contour, numbers, or time. These were common in subjects with Alzheimer's disease and Parkinson's disease with dementia and included unnecessary lines and writing letters. An example is shown in Figure 3-1B. Elaborations of the clock contour, defined as unnecessary additions to the contour such as a stand, were also seen, but this feature should not be considered pathological since it was seen in normals as well.

Although the proportion of the hands is frequently incorrect in patients with dementia, this feature alone is not useful for defining an abnormal response since many

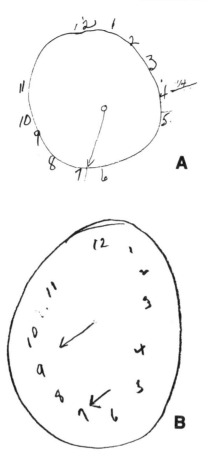

Figure 3–4   (A) Alzheimer's disease, female, age = 70 years. DRS = 102. (B) Parkinson's disease with dementia, female, age = 82 years, DRS = 111.

normals also have difficulty on this item, especially in the older age groups. In normals, even in their twenties, the frequency of occurrence of incorrect proportion is as high as 5 percent, and by the eighth decade the frequency reaches about 35 percent.

When two hands are drawn they are considered to be joined if the origins at the center are within a distance of 12 mm ($^1/_2$ in) from each other. Subjects with dementia who were able to draw two hands tended to join the hands as frequently as normals, although this was not always the case (Figure 3-4B).

In the subjects with Parkinson's disease without dementia, there were no statistically significant differences compared to normal controls on any of the critical items for hands. Subjects with low normal scores on the DRS, however, may still fail to draw two hands. This finding is very uncommon in normal subjects and should alert the clinician to the possibility of early cognitive impairment requiring further evaluation.

Center   Fewer patients with Alzheimer's disease and Parkinson's disease with dementia had a drawn or inferred center on their clocks, as compared to subjects without dementia. In cases in which there was a center, the subjects also tended to draw at least one hand, even though the hands did not always emanate from the drawn center. It is uncommon for patients with Alzheimer's disease or Parkinson's disease with dementia to place a dot in the center of the clock without subsequently drawing hands. We did not see any examples of this in our patients with dementia. We did, however, see this in one subject with Parkinson's disease who did not have dementia.

Subjects with Parkinson's disease without dementia were similar to normal subjects and tended to have a drawn or inferred center. Even the nondemented subject with Parkinson's disease in our series who did not place any hands on the clock still drew a center.

PRE-DRAWN CLOCKS (6:05)

Table 3-4 shows the performance profiles of the subjects on each of the critical items for numbers, hands, and center for the pre-drawn clock condition. In contrast to the free-drawn condition, the pre-drawn clock permits the assessment of number-drawing ability without the potentially confounding effects of a poorly drawn contour.

Numbers   The performance profile of the patients with Alzheimer's disease on the pre-drawn and free-drawn clocks was similar except that patients who do not rotate the paper on the free-drawn clock may do so on the pre-drawn clock. In our series, this occurred in two of the most severely impaired subjects. Also, in comparison to the free-drawn clocks, fewer patients with Parkinson's disease and dementia tended to place numbers outside the contour on the pre-drawn clocks. This may reflect the increased structure and reduced task demands of the pre-drawn clock compared to the free-drawn condition.

In the earlier stages of Alzheimer's disease, there was a relatively preserved ability to represent all 12 numbers and to space the numbers around the periphery of the clock contour. Patients may, however, still put in extra numbers and combine Roman with Arabic numerals on the clock face. Although the numbers tended to be in the correct sequence in the more mildly affected subjects, the position of the numbers was often incorrect.

Our findings suggest that as patients with Alzheimer's disease become more severely impaired they start to show a deterioration in the ability to place all of the numbers on the clock face and begin to space the numbers very poorly. Some patients tended to place the numbers in the right half of the clock, which raises the question of asymmetrical involvement affecting the right hemisphere of the brain more than the left (Figure 3-3B). Clocks drawn by patients with lesions in the right hemisphere are more fully discussed in Chapter 5. Also, the clock numbers may be located outside of the contour. In the more severely affected subjects there was a complete failure to draw any numbers at all. These patients may, however, attempt to write the numbers and the time on the clock face using a verbal strategy. The patient shown in Figure 3-5A attempted

TABLE 3-4. Pre-Drawn Clocks

	Percentage of Subjects with a Given Response[†]			
	AD (n=13)	DPD (n=14)	NDPD (n=20)	Normals (n=176)
Numbers				
Only numbers 1–12 present	30.8**	57.1**	80.0	92.6
Only Arabic numbers used	76.9**	92.9*	89.5 (n=19)	96.0
Numbers in correct order	83.3** (n=12)	92.3 (n=13)	100.0 (n=19)	99.4
Numbers drawn without rotating paper	83.3* (n=12)	100.0	100.0 (n=19)	94.9
Numbers in correct position	41.7** (n=12)	7.1**	84.2 (n=19)	77.3
Numbers inside contour	76.9	100.0	84.2 (n=19)	92.0
Hands				
Two hands present	46.2**	28.6**	85.0	94.3
Hour target number indicated	69.2**	71.4**	95.0*	100.0
Minute target number indicated	15.4**	21.4**	85.0	92.6
Hands in correct proportion	66.7 (n=6)	25.0 (n=4)	64.7 (n=17)	64.5 (n=166)
No superfluous markings	46.2**	64.3*	90.0	93.8
Hands relatively joined	83.3 (n=6)	100.0 (n=4)	100.0 (n=17)	97.0 (n=166)
Center				
Center is present (drawn or inferred)	53.8**	42.9**	95.0	94.9

[†] Percentage based only on subjects in whom the item could be scored. The sample size is shown in parentheses when less than original total.

* $p \leq 0.01$.

** $p \leq 0.001$.

to write a 12 at the top of the clock using letters and also tried to indicate the time by writing "five after 6" using a combination of incorrectly spelled words and a number.

Patients in the earlier stages of Parkinson's dementia demonstrated the ability to draw all 12 numbers. Even in the early stages, however, the position of the numbers tended to be very poor (Figure 3-5B). This was in contrast to the more mildly affected patients with Alzheimer's disease who tended to position their numbers better. The poorer positioning of the numbers in Parkinson's dementia may reflect difficulty with planning attributable to the prominent frontal system deficits in this disorder (Bowen et al., 1975; Cools et al., 1984; Flowers, 1982; Flowers & Robertson, 1985; Freedman & Oscar-Berman, 1986; Lees & Smith, 1983; Taylor et al., 1986). In contrast, early Alzheimer's disease is characterized by prominent deficits that are most marked in the temporoparietal regions as opposed to the frontal lobes (Brun & Englund, 1981; Chase, Foster, & Fedio, 1984; Cutler, Haxby, & Duara, 1985). As the subjects with Parkin-

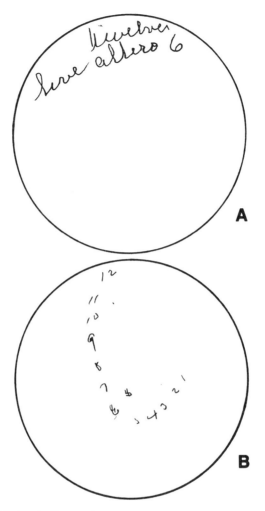

Figure 3–5   (A) Alzheimer's disease, female, age = 70 years, DRS = 71. (B) Parkinson's disease with dementia, female, age = 81 years, DRS = 121.

son's dementia become more severely impaired, our findings indicate that they begin to show errors characterized by number omission and more severe disorders of number position. Number additions and counterclockwise sequencing of the numbers also occurred. The most severely affected subjects drew no numbers at all.

In patients with Parkinson's disease without dementia, no significant differences existed in the performance profile compared to normal controls on the items related to numbers. The vast majority of patients with Parkinson's disease who were not demented placed all of the numbers on the clock without errors in sequence or position. In a small minority of Parkinson's patients without dementia, however, there were extra numbers, number omissions, and even complete failure to draw any numbers.

This tended to occur in subjects with DRS scores in the low normal range, and it again raises the question of cognitive dysfunction in this subgroup.

Hands Patients with Alzheimer's disease and Parkinson's disease with dementia were significantly impaired on most of the critical items for hands. Subjects with Alzheimer's disease who were mildly impaired were often able to place both hands on the clock and join the hands fairly well at the center. The proportion of the hands, however, was often incorrect. Although the hour hand was generally pointing to the correct number in the mildly affected subjects (e.g., for "6:05"), the minute hand tended to be drawn either to the "5" due to a stimulus-bound frontal pull, to another incorrect number such as the "12," or to a position between the "5" and the "6." One subject in our sample also drew a "spokes-of-a-wheel" pattern that is commonly seen after right-sided brain lesions (Figure 3-6A).

The more severely impaired patients with Alzheimer's disease did not draw any hands. If only one hand was drawn, this was almost always the hour hand. As described above, some subjects represented the time using a verbal strategy by writing the time across the clock face using words or in a digital fashion such as "605."

Similar to subjects with Alzheimer's disease, the majority of patients with Parkinson's dementia also failed to draw two hands. When two hands were drawn, however, there was a prominent tendency to draw the minute hand at the "5" or just after it. This likely represents the prominent frontal system deficits in Parkinson's dementia. Other examples of a concrete response were writing "65" across the clock face, drawing an extra "6" in the center of the clock and then drawing a line between the extra "6" and the "5," and placing a "6" and a "5" at the "6" and "1" positions, respectively. The latter response is shown in Figure 3-6B. In contrast to the minute hand, when the hour hand was drawn it tended to be targeted at the correct number.

Almost all subjects with Parkinson's disease without dementia were able to draw two hands and set the time correctly. The proportion of the hands was frequently incorrect but not more often than in normals. Some subjects, however, displayed signs suggestive of early frontal lobe deficits. One subject, for example, made a mark at the "6" and the "5" positions. These marks represent a strong pull to the numbers with a focus on the literal surface value. Other abnormal responses included a single hand pointing toward the hour target number, and a complete omission of hands. These types of responses were, however, uncommon in nondemented Parkinson's patients.

Center Significantly fewer patients with dementia due to Alzheimer's disease or Parkinson's disease had a drawn or inferred center on their pre-drawn clocks, as compared to subjects without dementia. In general, subjects drew a center only when there was at least one hand present.

EXAMINER CLOCKS

The examiner clock is useful for assessing the ability to draw the hands and center without the potentially confounding influence of a poor contour or abnormally drawn

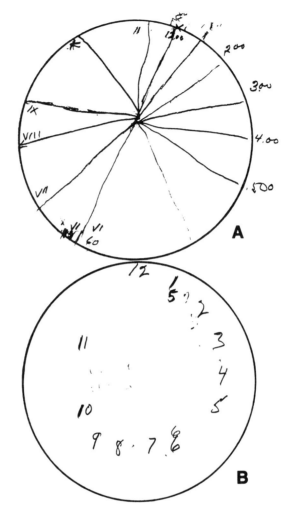

Figure 3–6   (A) Alzheimer's disease, male, age = 78 years, DRS = 122. (B) Parkinson's disease with dementia, female, age = 79 years, DRS = 121.

numbers. Tables 3-5, 3-6, and 3-7 show the performance profiles of the subjects on the critical items for hands and center.

Hands and Center   Patients with Alzheimer's disease and Parkinson's disease with dementia were significantly impaired on many of the critical items for hands at all three times, as well as on drawing the center on the three examiner clocks.

The ability to draw hands and to set the time accurately declined with increased severity of disease as measured by the DRS. In general, patients with Alzheimer's disease and Parkinson's disease with dementia who had a DRS greater than 100 were

TABLE 3-5. Examiner Clocks (11:10)

	Percentage of Subjects with a Given Response[†]			
	AD (n=13)	**DPD** (n=14)	**NDPD** (n=20)	**Normals** (n=176)
Hands				
Two hands present	53.8**	35.7**	85.0	93.8
Hour target number indicated	84.6**	92.9*	100.0	99.4
Minute target number indicated	15.4**	28.6**	85.0	93.8
Hands in correct proportion	66.7	40.0	82.4	78.2
	(n=6)	(n=5)	(n=17)	(n=165)
Hour hand/mark not displaced	58.3**	61.5	100.0	90.9
	(n=12)	(n=13)		
Minute hand/mark not displaced	37.5**	50.0	100.0	92.3
	(n=8)	(n=8)	(n=17)	(n=169)
No superfluous markings	46.2**	85.7	85.0	96.0
Hands relatively joined	100.0	80.0	100.0	97.6
	(n=7)	(n=5)	(n=17)	(n=165)
Center				
Center is present	61.5**	42.9**	90.0	92.6
Center is not displaced from vertical axis	87.5	75.0	94.1	94.5
	(n=8)	(n=4)	(n=17)	(n=163)
Center is not displaced from horizontal axis	75.0	50.0*	94.1	91.4
	(n=8)	(n=4)	(n=17)	(n=163)

[†] Percentage based only on subjects in whom the item could be scored. The sample size is shown in parentheses when less than original total.

* $p \leq 0.01$.

** $p \leq 0.001$.

able to draw an hour hand on examiner clocks regardless of the time setting. Displacement from the hour target number tended to occur more commonly for the "11:10" time setting than for the "8:20" or "3:00" setting.

Patients showed a striking difference in performance on drawing the minute hand depending on the time being set. The "11:10" and "8:20" time settings were more sensitive than the "3:00" setting to cognitive impairment. For the "11:10" setting, the instruction "10 minutes after" must be recoded as the numeral "2." Moreover, since the number "10" is located immediately adjacent to the "11," there is a tendency for subjects with frontal lobe impairment to be "pulled" to the "10" and to set the hands at "10" to "11." Similarly, for "8:20" the subject must recode the "20 minutes after 8" as the numeral "4." Some patients with frontal lobe deficits set the minute hand at the "2" because this number most closely resembles the "20." In contrast, a verbal recoding process is not required for "3:00" other than representing the "o'clock" by a "12."

The relative sensitivity of the time settings is well illustrated in Figure 3-7, which shows a classical frontal pull to the "10" for "10 after 11." The "8:20" clock shows one

TABLE 3-6.   Examiner Clocks (8:20)

	Percentage of Subjects with a Given Response[†]			
	AD (n=13)	DPD (n=14)	NDPD (n=20)	Normals (n=176)
Hands				
Two hands present	38.5**	28.6**	85.0	94.3
Hour target number indicated	92.3**	92.9*	95.0*	100.0
Minute target number indicated	23.1**	35.7**	85.0	94.3
Hands in correct proportion	60.0	75.0	76.5	77.7
	(n=5)	(n=4)	(n=17)	(n=166)
Hour hand/mark not displaced	91.7	84.6*	94.7	98.3
	(n=12)	(n=13)	(n=19)	
Minute hand/mark not displaced	50.0**	83.3	100.0	88.2
	(n=6)	(n=6)	(n=17)	(n=169)
No superfluous markings	25.0**	92.9	85.0**	97.2
	(n=12)			
Hands relatively joined	100.0	100.0	100.0	98.2
	(n=5)	(n=4)	(n=17)	(n=166)
Center				
Center is present	61.5**	35.7**	95.0	94.3
Center is not displaced from vertical axis	87.5	66.7	94.4	94.6
	(n=8)	(n=3)	(n=18)	(n=166)
Center is not displaced from horizontal axis	87.5	100.0	88.9	92.2
	(n=8)	(n=3)	(n=18)	(n=166)

[†] Percentage based only on subjects in whom the item could be scored. The sample size is shown in parentheses when less than original total.

* $p \leq 0.01$.

** $p \leq 0.001$.

hand at the "8" and another hand just "after" the "8." In contrast, the "3:00" time is set correctly although the proportion of the hands is incorrect. Figure 3-8A shows a typical frontal response for "8:20" where the subject is pulled to the "2" for the "20" and puts a mark at the "2." Figure 3-8B shows a typical frontal response that is seen in more severely impaired patients in which a "10" is placed after the "11" in a very concrete fashion. Such patients often place a "20" after the "8" for "8:20."

Other abnormal responses on the examiner clocks included joining the hour and minute target numbers by a straight line and superfluous markings. Superfluous markings included writing words on the clock face, drawing lines that are not hands, drawing circles within the clock face, and writing the time across the clock face using numbers. In some patients with dementia there was a displacement of the center toward the target numbers (Figure 3-7) but this was not a consistent finding.

The vast majority of patients with Parkinson's disease who were not demented drew hands and a center in a manner that was comparable to normals. Some Parkinson's patients without dementia who had DRS scores in the lower range of normal nevertheless did have impaired performances. The errors included drawing a single hand,

TABLE 3-7.   Examiner Clocks (3:00)

	Percentage of Subjects with a Given Response†			
	AD (n=13)	DPD (n=14)	NDPD (n=20)	Normals (n=176)
Hands				
Two hands present	46.2**	42.9**	95.0	94.3
Hour target number indicated	92.3**	85.7**	100.0	100.0
Minute target number indicated	30.8**	57.1**	95.0	97.2
Hands in correct proportion	33.3	33.3	68.4	74.1
	(n=6)	(n=6)	(n=19)	(n=166)
Hour hand/mark not displaced	92.3	91.7	95.0	96.6
		(n=12)		
Minute hand/mark not displaced	66.7	100.0	100.0	93.0
	(n=6)	(n=8)	(n=19)	(n=171)
No superfluous markings	46.2**	92.9*	90.0*	98.9
Hands relatively joined	100.0	100.0	100.0	97.6
	(n=6)	(n=6)	(n=19)	(n=166)
Center				
Center is present	61.5**	42.9**	95.0	94.3
Center is not displaced from vertical axis	100.0	80.0	88.9	92.8
	(n=8)	(n=5)	(n=18)	(n=166)
Center is not displaced from horizontal axis	87.5	100.0	94.4	97.6
	(n=8)	(n=5)	(n=18)	(n=166)

† Percentage based only on subjects in whom the item could be scored. The sample size is shown in parentheses when less than original total.

* $p \leq 0.01$.

** $p \leq 0.001$.

failing to indicate any target numbers, drawing superfluous markings such as a small "20" beside the "4" on an "8:20" clock, and making a mark after the "11" and "8" on the "11:10" and "8:20" clocks, respectively. Similarly to the subjects with dementia, there were some patients who drew a center that was displaced toward the target numbers.

Summary of Clock Drawing in Dementia

Clock drawing has been shown to be a sensitive measure of cognitive impairment in patients with dementia due to different causes, including Alzheimer's disease, Parkinson's disease, Huntington's disease, and multi-infarct dementia. Although there are a variety of different methods of administration and scoring, significant abnormalities have been demonstrated on free-drawn, pre-drawn, and examiner clocks. The deficits are reflected in total clock scores, as well as in selective components of the clock-drawing task. As would be expected, patients with more severe dementia show more deficits on clock drawing as compared to those with mild impairment. This is clearly

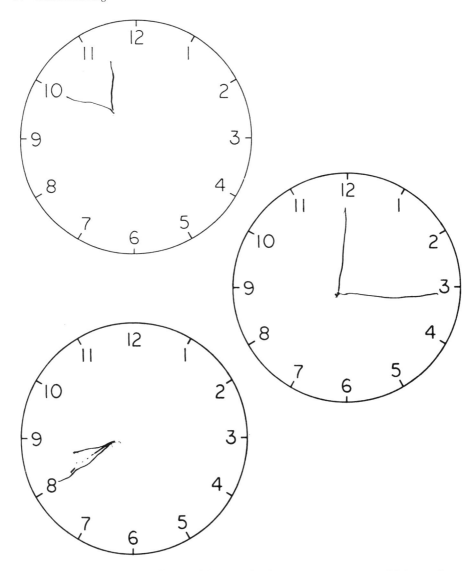

Figure 3–7   Parkinson's disease with dementia, female, age = 74 years, DRS = 113.

demonstrated in the longitudinal follow-up of patients with dementia. Figure 3-9A shows a clock drawn by a female patient in the early stages of Alzheimer's disease. Although the final production is correct, the process by which the clock was drawn is disorganized and the patient made several errors that she was able to self-correct. Figure 3-9B shows a clock drawn by the same patient 14 months later when she no longer had the capacity to correct her errors.

The abnormalities on the critical items from our normative study that were charac-

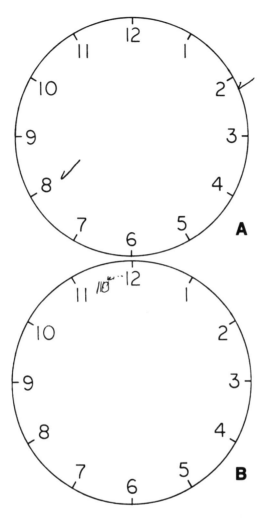

Figure 3–8   (A) Alzheimer's disease, female, age = 68 years, DRS = 95. (B) Alzheimer's disease, female, age = 73 years, DRS = 86.

teristic of impaired clock drawing in patients with Alzheimer's disease and Parkinson's disease with dementia included drawing poor contours, omission of numbers, adding extra numbers, placing numbers in the incorrect order, failing to draw two hands, poor placement of the minute hand, inability to indicate accurately the hour hand, and drawing superfluous markings (excluding strokes demarcating the 5-minute intervals). Other abnormal responses indicative of dementia included writing the minutes (e.g., "10") next to the hour target number, writing the time on the clock face literally (e.g., "605"), a frontal pull for the minute hand such as drawing the hands at "10" to "11" rather than "10" after "11," and inability to draw numbers. These findings are in keeping with those of others who documented drawing irrelevant figures such as

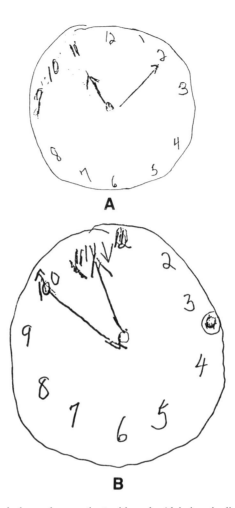

A

B

Figure 3–9 (A) A clock drawn by a patient with early Alzheimer's disease. She wrote in the numbers "12," "3," "6," and "9" in the four quadrants, wrote in "10" and "11," set one hand for "11," drew the center dot, wrote in "1," "2," "4," and "5," set a second hand on "10" (a stimulus-bound response), erased this hand and set it on "2," wrote in "8" and "7," erased the "3" and rewrote it, erased the "9," "10," and "11" and rewrote them, and erased the hand set for "11" and drew it shorter. (B) A clock drawn by the same patient as in Figure 9A 14 months later. She wrote in "11" at the top, "4" on the right, and "10" in the upper left quadrant, wrote in "2" and "3," crossed out the "4," wrote "4," "5," "6," "9," "7," "8," another "10," two "11's," and "12," set the hands for "10 to 11" (with spatial reversal of one hand), and perseverated in drawing extra hands near the "10" and "11."

words, irrelevant spatial arrangement of the numbers, counterclockwise rotation, failure to draw any numbers, perseveration, writing numbers outside the clocks, and omission and misplacement of numbers (Rouleau et al., 1992; Sunderland et al., 1989; Tuokko et al., 1992; Wolf-Klein et al., 1989). Differences also have been found between different types of dementia. For example, patients with Alzheimer's disease tend to draw larger clocks to command compared to those with Huntington's disease.

Metabolic Encephalopathy

Metabolic encephalopathy is caused by endogenous toxins (e.g., uremia, hepatic insufficiency), exogenous toxins (e.g., heavy metals, alcohol), and endogenous hormone deficiency (e.g., hypothyroidism) (Cummings & Benson, 1983). These disorders may result in peripheral neuropathy and widespread involvement of different brain regions. For example, the lesions in Wernicke's encephalopathy secondary to thiamine deficiency in alcoholics typically include damage in the thalamus and hypothalamus, mamillary bodies, midbrain, pons, medulla, and vermis of the cerebellum (Victor, 1979).

A common sequela of metabolic encephalopathy is anterograde amnesia (Butters & Cermak, 1980). The tendency to make perseverative intrusion errors often occurs in amnesia, especially in acute stages when confusion is present (Figure 3-10A). Hand tremor will be revealed in wavy lines (Figure 3-10C,D). Visuospatial disorganization is also common (Figure 3-10C–E). In severe cases, cognitive deficits associated with frontal system dysfunction are also seen such as stimulus-bound responses (Figure 3-10C,D) and perseveration (Figure 3-10A,B,E).

Traumatic Brain Injury

Traumatic brain injuries (TBI) range from mild concussion with brief loss of consciousness (seconds to minutes) without demonstrable neurological findings, to severe injury with long periods of unconsciousness (weeks to months), abnormal neurologic signs, and cerebral contusion, edema, and laceration (Levin, Benton, & Grossman, 1982). When permanent injury has occurred, the neuropsychological sequelae will depend on the nature, site, and severity of the trauma. Brain structures that are particularly vulnerable to head trauma are the brain stem, the frontal, temporal, and occipital poles, and periventricular structures. Superimposed on these general sites of involvement are those areas in which focal damage (contusion or hemorrhage) occurs. The focal damage may occur directly at the site of the trauma's impact and/or contralateral to the zone of impact (i.e., the contrecoup injury; Levin et al., 1982).

With bifrontal contusions, mild deficits associated with frontal lobe dysfunction may be the only finding (e.g., a stimulus-bound time setting; Figure 3-11A). Brain stem and periventricular involvement from severe head trauma frequently results in micrographia and spatial problems in addition to the classical "frontal" deficits (Figure 3-11B–E). Depending on the location of the focal involvement, different combinations of spatial and number-writing deficits will occur (Figure 3-11E,F).

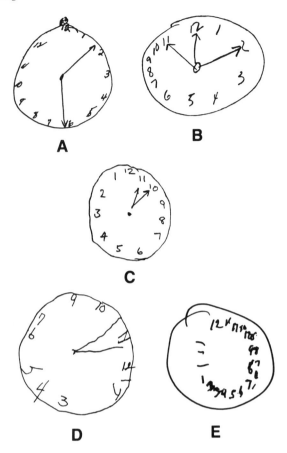

Figure 3–10   Clocks drawn by patients with metabolic encephalopathy illustrating
(A) inability to maintain the correct spatial layout while sequencing the numbers, and
perseveration of an extra "12" (in a patient with alcoholic Korsakoff syndrome); (B) inability
to remember if the time setting was "11 o'clock" or "10 after 11" (in a patient with alcoholic
dementia); (C) mirror reversal of number placement and stimulus-bound time setting (in a
patient with subacute hepatic encephalopathy); (D) 90-degree rotation of number sequence
and stimulus-bound time setting (in a patient with inorganic mercury poisoning); and
(E) incorrect number sequence, inability to maintain correct spatial layout while sequencing
numbers, omission of hands, and perseveration of extra numbers (in a patient with cognitive
impairment secondary to chronic obstructive pulmonary disease).

Disconnection Syndrome

The clock-drawing task can be used in assessing disconnection in split-brain syndromes. The clocks shown in Figure 3-12 were drawn by a patient who suffered a
cerebral infarct in the left posterior cerebral artery territory. This lesion typically
damages the left occipital lobe and the posterior portion of the corpus callosum (the

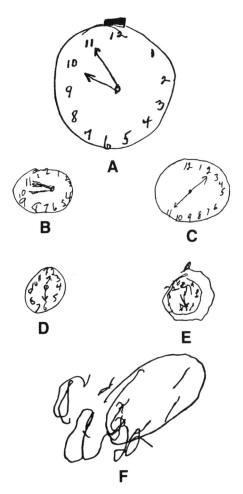

Figure 3–11   Clocks drawn by patients with mild to severe head trauma illustrating
(A) stimulus-bound time setting (in a patient with mild bifrontal contusions); (B) stimulus-
bound time setting, micrographia, and overwriting of hands (in a patient with ventricular
enlargement); (C) inability to maintain the correct spatial layout while sequencing the
numbers (in a patient with bifrontal hemorrhage); (D) micrographia, incorrect time setting,
and a possible confusion of "12" as "1" and "2" (in a patient with a left frontotemporal
subdural hematoma); (E) micrographia, agraphia, poor fine-motor control, perseveration of
clock face and incorrect time setting (in patient with bifrontal subdural hematoma); and
(F) severe spatial disorganization and numerical agraphia (in a patient with a residual large
left frontal lesion and small right frontal-parietal lesion).

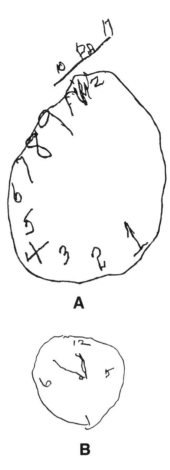

A

B

Figure 3–12   Clocks drawn to command by a patient with damage to the left occipital lobe and posterior portion of the corpus callosum (the splenium); the patient displayed the disconnection syndrome of alexia without agraphia. Clock (A) drawn with his right hand (and primarily left hemisphere) illustrates preserved number sequencing, but spatial disorientation of the sequence, displacement of the one hand outside the clock, and reliance on a verbal strategy to represent "10 after 11." Clock (B), drawn with his left hand (and primarily right hemisphere), is spatially more coherent, with numbers included at all four quadrants and both hands present; however, number sequencing is severely impaired, eight of the numbers are omitted, and the time setting is inaccurate (which may reflect verbal comprehension or memory problems).

splenium). As a result, visual information can be projected only to the occipital lobe in the right hemisphere, and it cannot cross over to the language areas in the left hemisphere due to the damage to the splenium. Patients with this type of damage often present with "alexia without agraphia," a disconnection syndrome characterized by an inability to read with preserved writing ability (Geschwind, 1965; Geschwind & Kaplan, 1962).

The patient shown in Figure 3-12 incurred damage to only the posterior part of his corpus callosum. Would his disconnection syndrome be revealed on other tasks besides reading that involved the visual modality? To address this question the patient was asked to draw the clocks twice. Figure 3-12A,B shows the patient's drawings to command with his right and left hand, respectively. With his right hand he drew the clock with all the numbers in the correct sequence but the spatial layout of the sequence within the clock face was incorrect. After writing in the numbers, he drew only one hand outside the clock face, which also reflected spatial disorganization. In addition, he relied on a verbal strategy to represent the time setting by writing "10 pa 11" on the single clock hand. Thus, when using his right hand, the patient did not appear to benefit from the global spatial functions that presumably would be mediated by his intact right hemisphere.

When the patient drew the clock with his left hand, a qualitatively different clock emerged (Figure 3-12B). He constructed the clock face and the two hands before attempting to write the numbers. The hands were drawn in a spatially appropriate manner, although they were set for 11 o'clock instead of "10 after 11." This incorrect time setting may reflect a verbal memory deficit secondary to his mesial left posterior damage or a language comprehension problem because he was working with his left hand (and predominantly right hemisphere). The patient then drew in only four numbers. Two of the four numbers were out of sequence, but the four numbers were placed in a spatially organized array (i.e., at 90°, 180°, 270°, and 360° positions).

Thus with his right hand (and presumably greater use of the left hemisphere), this patient generated the correct sequence of numbers but oriented the numbers and the one hand in a disorganized manner. With his left hand, and presumably greater use of the right hemisphere (he constructed a spatially coherent clock with two hands but he omitted or incorrectly sequenced the numbers). All of the component cognitive functions necessary to draw a clock were manifested in one drawing or the other, but the processes remained disconnected.

Clock Drawing in Dementia: Longitudinal Follow-up

One of the authors of this text (K. S.), together with Dr. Dolores Gold and Dr. Carole Cohen (Shulman, Gold, Cohen, and Zucchero, 1993), incorporated clock drawing into a battery of instruments to study a group of dementing patients and their caregivers. We had a unique opportunity to evaluate its sensitivity to cognitive change over time. We compared clock drawing to other standardized and well-validated tests of mental status and global functioning.

Because we were following a group of patients who were expected to show progressive cognitive decline, we hoped to confirm prior clinical impressions that clock drawing was indeed sensitive to change in mental function. If this proved to be the case, the test could be a useful and practical adjunct for clinicians who need assessment instruments that are quick and easy to administer and are not unduly influenced by educational or cultural factors.

The study was designed to examine psychosocial factors that influence a caregiver's decision to institutionalize or maintain dependents in the community. The following criteria were used to select patients with dementia and their caregivers for investigation: (1) patients diagnosed as suffering from dementia according to DSM-III criteria and who had experienced a progressive dementia for at least one year and did not have another psychiatric syndrome that could account for the dementia; (2) the patients had resided at home with no extended absences during the past year; and (3) patients had at least one caregiver, a relative or friend, who provided regular and essential care and support. These were the patients included in the study. Patients with an active and disabling medical condition of a severity that threatened their physical independence were excluded. Patients were also excluded if there was evidence of gross visual impairment that could interfere with clock drawing.

Complete data were available for the following numbers of patients at four points in time: 183 at initial assessment, 111 at 6-month follow-up, 56 at 12 months, and 19 at 18 months. At initial assessment, the patients had a mean age of 77.5 ± 8.1 years and a mean educational level of 11.4 ± 3.7 years. Home care had been continuing for a mean duration of 3.3 ± 2.7 years.

The primary caregivers were asked a series of questions at each assessment, ascertaining their commitment to continuing home care. Specifically, they were asked whether they would continue to care for their relative at home or place the person in an institution, assuming that satisfactory residential care was immediately available. At the four assessment periods, a total of 142, 78, 52, and all of the 19 remaining participating caregivers had decided to continue home care, whereas the rest of the participating caregivers had decided to end home care.

The measures of cognitive function that were included in the battery were the Mini-Mental State Examination (Folstein, Folstein, & McHugh, 1975), a revised and shortened Clifton Assessment Schedule (Pattie & Gilleard, 1975), and the Global Deterioration Scale (Reisberg, Ferris, De Leon et al., 1982). A list of empirically derived psychiatric symptoms was compiled as part of the initial and 6-month psychiatric evaluation. Data collected for each patient included basic demographic information such as age, sex, socioeconomic, ethnic and marital status, personal and family history, and characteristics of residence. A random reliability check of approximately 25 percent of the sample was carried out.

All patients were presented with a pre-drawn circle and given the instruction to "Put the numbers on the clock and set the time at 10 after 11."

Clock scores decreased with time due to overall deterioration of function, but the relation of these scores between patients remained consistent across time at initial, 6-month, 12-month, and 18-month assessments. Table 3-8 provides a measure of test-retest reliability. In the normative chapter, the measures of the test-retest reliability were low owing to the limited range of scores of the normal subjects. The average coefficient across subsequent administration of clock drawing in the present study yielded a test-retest correlation of .89.

All tests showed the predicted pattern of deterioration in cognition over time. One particularly interesting result of this study revealed that the only measure associated

TABLE 3-8. Correlation Coefficients for Clock Drawing Across Assessments*

	Clock Scores		
Clock Scores	6 Month	12 Month	18 Month
Initial	.85	.84	.89
6 Month		.89	.90
12 Month			.95

* All coefficients at $p < 0.001$.

with the caregiver's decision to end home care was the difference on the clock scores. Univariate ANOVAs found only the clock score differences to be associated with the outcome described, $F(1,103) = 4.09$, $p < .05$. That is, those dependents whose caregivers indicated at initial assessment that they intended to institutionalize showed the greatest decline in clock scores. Moreover, those same dependents with significant decline in clock scores were in fact institutionalized at a higher rate at follow-up.

QUALITATIVE CHANGES OVER TIME

The types of errors that were seen include organizational problems, impairment in abstract ability, and ultimately a complete inability to understand and execute the functions required for clock drawing. We shall highlight those patients whose clocks showed obvious decline over the 6- to 18-month follow-up period. Figures 3-13 through 3-16 show a number of examples of this type of deterioration over time.

Figure 3-13 shows three patients whose initial assessment revealed an advanced level of deterioration in clock drawing. In all three cases within the 6-month to 12-month follow-up assessments, no attempt at all was possible at clock drawing because of the severe deterioration in cognition. Thus, the only documentation is a virtually empty circle as demonstrated in each of these three cases.

Figure 3-14 shows four patients whose initial clock drawing showed a moderate level of impairment with severe visuospatial disorganization. They exhibited a similar progression to an eventual stage of complete inability to draw a clock. However, the moderately impaired group appeared to take somewhat longer (from 12 to 18 months) before reaching that stage where they are incapable of drawing any features of a clock.

Figure 3-15 shows clocks that were drawn with relatively intact visuospatial organization, but the patients were unable to denote "10 after 11" as per the usual instruction. These patients eventually all progressed to obvious impairment, but importantly were unable to use hands at all during the follow-up period. This confirms our intuitive impression that the inability to denote accurate time (i.e., "10 after 11") by the use of hands is a significant indication of cognitive impairment and should be seen as a more serious error than visuospatial difficulties.

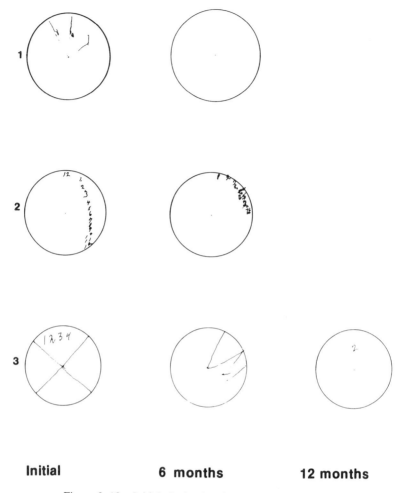

Initial   **6 months**   **12 months**

Figure 3–13   Initial clocks showing severe deterioration.

In Figure 3-16, patients showed a normal ability to draw clocks at the initial assessment. However, in dementing patients this ability was not sustained. In the three
cases shown in Figure 3-16, the patients all went on to progressive decline in clock-
drawing ability. At 6 months, Patient 1 shows the visuospatial organization to be less
precise, with numbers showing greater distance from the clock border and the patient
has omitted the minute hand in the follow-up clock. Patient 2 went on to show more
severe visuospatial disorganization within a 6-month period. Patient 3 invites some
controversy. A "perfect" clock at initial assessment shows more subtle changes at 6
months such as moving numbers beyond the clock border and then reverting to Roman
numerals at 12 months. It is uncertain whether this represents a form of "regression"
in clock drawing, because all numbers were correctly placed and the time set was cor-

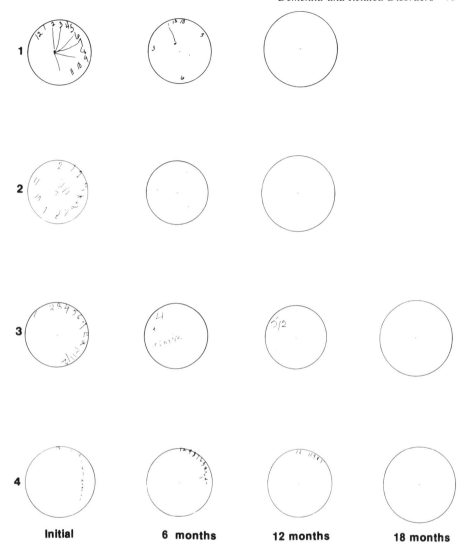

| | **Initial** | **6 months** | **12 months** | **18 months** |

Figure 3–14   Initial clocks showing moderate deterioration.

rect. Nevertheless, this particular patient was institutionalized 6 months after the last follow-up.

To summarize, we found that clock-drawing ability deteriorated in parallel with cognitive and functional status. Furthermore, of the measures used in this study, clock drawing was shown to be the best that would predict whether or not an individual would require institutionalization. This indicates that a clock-drawing test can be a useful adjunct for clinicians who must monitor dementing individuals in order to help caregivers make decisions regarding institutionalization.

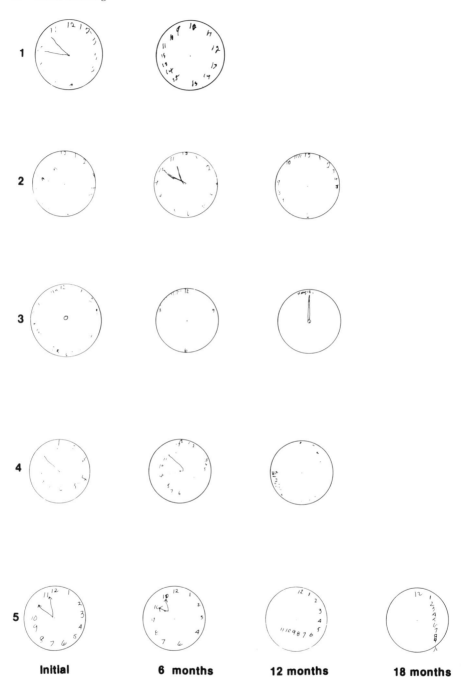

Figure 3–15   Initial clocks with impairment of denoting time.

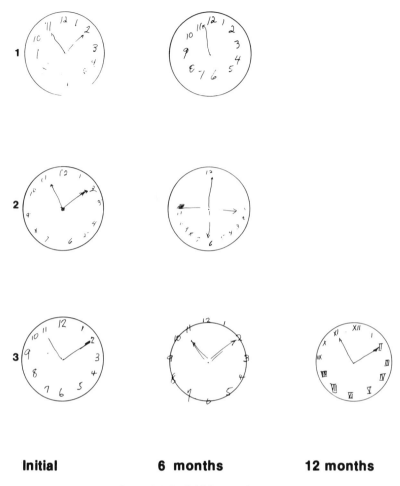

Initial   **6 months**   **12 months**

Figure 3–16   Initial normal clocks.

Conclusions

Clock drawing is sensitive to cognitive deficits resulting from dementia and related disorders such as metabolic encephalopathy, traumatic brain injury, and disconnection syndromes. Although the different clock conditions (i.e., free-drawn, pre-drawn, and examiner) have features in common, they differ in the clinical information they provide. If only one condition can be administered, we suggest that the free-drawn clock be selected. It is the only condition that contains all of the elements of the clock-drawing task. The assessment of contour is very important as a screening item since the inability to draw an acceptable contour can be considered pathological at any age. The free-drawn clock allows for the assessment of numbers, but this may be confounded by a poor contour. Similarly, drawing the hands and center may be affected by both a poor contour and impaired drawing of the numbers. The pre-drawn clock, on the other hand, is useful for assessing the ability to draw numbers, hands, and the center. The examiner clock is best for assessing the ability to place the hands and center on the clock. Ideally, all three clock conditions should be administered.

On the examiner clocks, the ability of the patient to draw the hands differed according to the time setting requested. Times that require a recoding of the literal value of the minute hand are most sensitive for demonstrating cognitive deficits, particularly frontal system abnormalities. The "11:10" and "8:20" time settings are, therefore, more sensitive than the "3:00" setting. Even for the "11:10" and "8:20" times, however, the types of responses differ. The classical frontal pull to the minute target number is seen for "11:10," where the minute hand is drawn toward the "10," which is situated right beside the "11." For "8:20," there is no "20" on the clock to "pull" the subjects and so other abnormal responses tend to occur such as placement of the minute hand just after the "8" or drawing a minute hand toward the "2" because of its resemblance to a "20."

Finally, it is important to stress that although clock drawing is a sensitive screening measure for cognitive impairment, this task is not intended to serve as a diagnostic tool for any specific type of disorder such as Alzheimer's disease. Instead, it serves to demonstrate deficits due to dysfunction in specific brain systems that may be affected by a broad spectrum of neurological disorders.

ACKNOWLEDGMENTS

The longitudinal study described in this chapter was carried out in collaboration with Dr. Dolores P. Gold, Department of Psychology, Concordia University, Montreal, Quebec, and Dr. Carole Cohen, Department of Psychiatry, Sunnybrook Health Science Centre, Toronto, Ontario, Canada.

4. Well Elderly in a Seniors' Residence

In previous chapters we described the clocks drawn by normal subjects, as well as by patients with dementia and related disorders. Falling outside these categories are a large number of elderly individuals who are functioning relatively well intellectually but who require assistance because of mild physical problems or social isolation. In many cases, they are unable to manage adequately without some degree of medical, nursing, and social support in a structured environment. Although some of these people may have early dementia, cognitive impairment is generally not their salient problem. Winocur and Moscovitch (1990), however, found that these individuals may show mild deficits on a variety of tasks that are sensitive to specific aspects of brain function. They administered a series of neuropsychological tests to persons living in institutions but who were free of known neurological, psychiatric, or serious physical disorders involving heart, lung, liver, and kidney function. Subjects had entered the institutions for reasons such as death of a spouse, family moving away, financial worries, or finding it difficult to live independently. There was no evidence of poor mental health. Nevertheless, they were found to have significant deficits on neuropsychological measures thought to be sensitive to frontal lobe and medial temporal lobe function. Although the battery of tests did not include clock drawing, clinical experience suggests that this task may also be sensitive to the cognitive deficits in the institutionalized well elderly.

In this chapter we shall describe clock-drawing ability in subjects living in a seniors' residence. In addition, we shall relate their clock-drawing ability to their performance on measures of general cognitive function. This will provide an important perspective on the significance of clock drawing as an indicator of early dementia. Moreover, this type of information will be helpful for the development of screening tests that utilize clock drawing as part of the entry assessment for seniors' residences and related institutions.

Because there are no data in the literature on clock drawing in the well elderly living in institutions, we shall focus on the findings from our own subjects living at Baycrest Terrace in Toronto, a seniors' residence offering on-site medical, nursing, and social support. There were 25 subjects who were between the ages of 72 and 90 years (mean 83.5 ± 4.9 years). Their level of education ranged from 6 to 16 years (mean 9.3 ± 2.6 years). Eighty-eight percent were female. All were able to manage independently in their apartments at the residence. None had a history of alcoholism, significant psychiatric disease, severe systemic disease, or neurological disorder.

Because the subjects at Baycrest Terrace were tested prior to our planning the normative study, the procedures differed in some respects from those described in Chapter 2. In the Baycrest Terrace sample, clock-drawing ability was assessed using three separate free-drawn conditions and three examiner clock conditions, as described below. General level of cognitive function was assessed with the Mattis Dementia Rating Scale (DRS) (Coblentz, Mattis, Zingesser, Kasoff, Wisniewski, & Katzman, 1973; Mattis, 1988). The Raven's Coloured Progressive Matrices provided a measure of nonverbal intelligence (Raven, 1965).

Free-Drawn Clock Condition

Subjects were presented with a blank sheet of 8½-by-11-inch white paper and given the following instructions: "I would like you to draw a clock and put in all the numbers." After the subject had done this the examiner said, "Now I would like you to set the time at 10 after 11." Subjects were then presented with a second blank sheet of paper and instructed to draw a clock and to set the hands at "20 after 8." Next, they were given a third sheet and asked to draw a clock and set the hands at "3 o'clock."

After completing the free-drawn clock condition, all subjects were administered the Raven's Coloured Progressive Matrices and the Dementia Rating Scale (DRS).

Examiner Clock Condition

Two to five months later, subjects were seen a second time and given three examiner clock conditions. For each condition, subjects were presented with a sheet of 8½-by-11-inch blank white paper with a pre-drawn, numbered clock face on it. The diameter was 8.5 cm (3⅜ in). The height of the numbers was 6 mm (¼ in). This contrasts with the normative study in which the clock face was 11.7 cm (4⅝ in) in diameter and the numbers were 7 mm (⁵⁄₁₆ in) high. As in the normative study, however, the examiner instructed the subjects to "Set the time at 10 after 11," "20 after 8," and "3 o'clock" in a counterbalanced order.

Because the DRS had been administered during the initial assessment for the free-drawn clock condition, it was given a second time only if more than four months had elapsed since the first administration. For the free-drawn clock condition, 6 of the 25 subjects obtained a DRS score of less than 123, which is the cutoff score we used for defining subjects as demented (Montgomery & Costa, 1983). After the subjects were seen a second time for assessment on the examiner clock condition, 11 required a second administration of the DRS because of the elapsed time. Two of these 11 subjects had DRS scores that changed from being above the cutoff for dementia to falling below 123. This resulted in a total of 8 of the 25 subjects falling within the "demented range" by the time the study had been completed. All of these subjects, however, were able to manage independently in their apartments and did not appear demented to the Baycrest Terrace staff. The range of DRS scores was 113–122 in the subgroup below the cutoff and 123–140 in the subgroup above the cutoff.

The free-drawn and examiner clocks produced by the Baycrest Terrace subjects were compared on the critical items outlined in the normative chapter (see Table 2-2). For each free-drawn clock a "total score" was calculated using the critical items for clock contour, numbers, hands, and center (maximum score, 15). The total score for each examiner clock was based upon the critical items dealing with hands and center (maximum score, 11).

We compared the clocks drawn by the Baycrest Terrace residents to those drawn by a representative sample of control subjects from the normative study who were living in the community. Both groups were equated for age and gender. As indicated above, subjects in the Baycrest Terrace group were tested prior to the plans for the normative study. Subjects in the Baycrest Terrace and in the community had both received the same initial instructions for the free-drawn clock condition, as follows: "I would like you to draw a clock and put in the numbers." The administration then differed for the time setting. Baycrest Terrace subjects had been asked to set the time at "10 after 11," "20 after 8," and "3 o'clock," respectively, whereas the normal elderly living in the community had been asked to produce only one free-drawn clock and to set the time at "a quarter to 7" according to the standard protocol outlined in the normative chapter. Owing to this difference in administration, the first free-drawn clock produced by the subjects in Baycrest Terrace was compared to the "6:45" free-drawn clock produced by the community elderly only for those items related to clock contour and numbers. No comparison was made for the hands or center since the time settings were different. The maximum total clock score on the free-drawn condition was, therefore, 8 rather than 15 as in the normative study. In contrast to the free-drawn clock, administration of the examiner clocks was identical for both the Baycrest Terrace and the community dwelling elderly.

Table 4-1 shows the mean total clock scores obtained by the subject groups on the

TABLE 4-1.   Total Clock Score

	Baycrest Terrace Elderly (n=25)		Community Dwelling Elderly (n=25)		
	Mean	**(SD)**	**Mean**	**(SD)**	***p***
Free-Drawn Clock	7.08	(.81)	7.56	(.65)	$p < .05$*
Examiner Clock					
(max score=11)					
11:10	8.44	(2.93)	8.76	(2.88)	NS
8:20	8.92	(2.80)	9.28	(2.68)	NS
3:00	9.28	(2.07)	9.28	(2.49)	NS

* Wilcoxon test (two-tailed).

free-drawn and examiner clock conditions, as well as a statistical comparison between the subject groups on the different clock conditions. There was a slight but statistically significant impairment of the Baycrest Terrace group on the free-drawn clock. No significant differences appeared on the examiner clocks.

Tables 4-2 and 4-3 show the quantitative data characterizing the performance profile of the Baycrest Terrace subjects and normal elderly on the critical items of the free-drawn and examiner clocks, respectively. Quantitative analysis, however, yielded little information that distinguished these relatively high-functioning groups. The major difference between the groups on the free-drawn clocks was the poor positioning of the numbers in the Baycrest Terrace subjects. Whereas 68 percent of normal subjects positioned the numbers correctly, only 36 percent of Baycrest Terrace subjects were able to do so ($p < .05$). Because position errors occurred in both groups, however, this type of error by itself should not be considered pathological. Severity of the poor positioning, on the other hand, may provide important information about the presence of cognitive impairment. This is illustrated in Figure 4-1, which shows incorrect positioning of the numbers in Baycrest Terrace subjects (Figure 4-1A,B) and normal controls (Figure 4-1C,D). The clocks drawn by the Baycrest Terrace subjects show a much poorer number placement as compared to the clocks drawn by normal controls. Moreover, the DRS scores of the Baycrest Terrace subjects were less than 123 in each of the two cases shown (i.e., in the impaired range). Figure 4-1D illustrates a markedly abnormal clock drawn by a normal control (female, age 81) that not only shows poor positioning of the numbers but also other deficits including superfluous markings in a "Christmas tree" pattern and inability to set the time. A "4" and "5" are placed before the "7" in a very literal response to "6:45," which is suggestive of frontal system dysfunction.

TABLE 4-2.   Free-Drawn Clocks

	Percentage of Subjects with a Given Response	
	Baycrest Terrace Subjects (n=25)	Controls (n=25)
Contour		
Attempted	100.0	100.0
Acceptable	100.0	100.0
Numbers		
Only numbers 1–12 present	88.0	96.0
Arabic number representation	100.0	96.0
Numbers in correct sequence	92.0	100.0
Numbers drawn without rotating paper	92.0	100.0
Numbers in correct position	36.0	68.0
Numbers inside contour	100.0	96.0

TABLE 4-3.   Examiner Clocks

	Percentage of Subjects with a Given Response*					
	Baycrest Terrace Residents (n=25)			Normal Controls (n=25)		
	11:10	8:20	3:00	11:10	8:20	3:00
Hands						
Two hands present	84	84	92	80	80	80
Hour target number indicated	96	100	100	100	100	100
Minute target number indicated	84	88	92	80	84	88
Hands in correct proportion	62	66.7	56.5	55	85	60
	(n=21)	(n=21)	(n=23)	(n=20)	(n=20)	(n=20)
Hour hand/mark not displaced	80	96	79	80	100	96
		(n=24)	(n=24)			
Minute hand/mark not	91	95	91	90	90	100
displaced	(n=22)	(n=22)	(n=22)	(n=21)	(n=21)	(n=22)
No superfluous markings	84	92	96	100	88	100
Hands relatively joined	95.2	100	100	100	100	95
	(n=21)	(n=21)	(n=23)	(n=20)	(n=20)	(n=20)
Center						
Center is present (drawn or inferred)	80	84	92	84	88	88
Center is not displaced from	67	80	78	90.5	100	90.9
the vertical axis	(n=21)	(n=20)	(n=23)	(n=21)	(n=22)	(n=22)
Center is not displaced from	76	80	91	90	86	95
the horizontal axis	(n=21)	(n=20)	(n=23)	(n=21)	(n=22)	(n=22)

* Percentage based only on subjects in whom the item could be scored. The sample size is shown in parentheses when less than the original total.

On the examiner clocks, the Baycrest Terrace subjects drew significantly more superfluous markings (e.g., Figure 4-2) on the "10 after 11" clock compared to the elderly in the community ($p < .05$).

Although pooling the clocks in the Baycrest Terrace group for comparison to elderly in the community is important for obtaining an overall perspective, combining the Baycrest Terrace subjects into a single group may obscure important information about the types of abnormal clocks that may be seen within subgroups of individuals. Because the majority of the poorly drawn clocks were produced by subjects with lower DRS scores, we compared the clocks drawn by the subjects with DRS scores of less than 123 (i.e., the cutoff for dementia) to those drawn by the subjects with scores of 123 or higher. We shall refer to the group with DRS scores of less than 123 as the low DRS (LoDRS) subgroup and the other group as the high DRS (HiDRS) subgroup. We should emphasize, however, that even the subjects with low DRS scores apparently were functioning adequately in the Terrace.

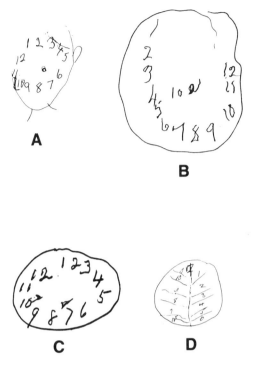

Figure 4–1   (A) Terrace subject; DRS 119, age 89; poor number placement, poor contour, and a curved line with a small arrowhead going from the 10 to the 11 for the hands placement. (B) Terrace subject, DRS 107, age 89; poor number placement with counterclockwise sequence. Also, the number 10 is written on the clock face for 11:10. (C) Normal control showing a representative example of poor number placement in this group, age 88. (D) Normal control showing unusual example of poor number placement and unusual superfluous markings in a "Christmas tree" pattern, age 81.

Free-Drawn Clock Condition

Table 4-4 shows total clock scores of the HiDRS and LoDRS Baycrest Terrace subjects and illustrates the significant group differences found on both the free-drawn and examiner clocks. Table 4-5 shows the performance profiles on each of the critical items for the free-drawn clock.

CONTOUR

All of the subjects from the Baycrest Terrace residence were able to draw an acceptable contour. Although the shapes tended to be more circular and symmetrical in the clocks drawn by the subjects in the HiDRS subgroup, considerable variability and overlap existed between the two subgroups. This is well illustrated in Figure 4-3, which shows a relatively good and poor contour in each of the LoDRS (Figure 4-3A,B) and HiDRS

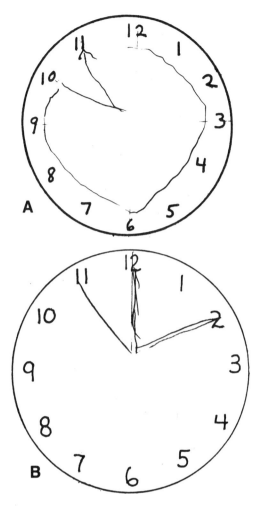

Figure 4–2   Superfluous markings on "10 after 11" clock in Terrace subjects: (A) Circular hand sweeping around inside the boundary of the clock. This clock also shows a frontal "pull" of the minute hand to the 10; DRS 113, age 79. (B) Third hand on clock; DRS 126, age 84.

(Figure 4-3C,D) subgroups. In a screening test for admission to a seniors' residence, therefore, all acceptable applicants should be able to draw a clock contour. The shape of the contour, however, may not be related to the ability to function independently.

NUMBERS

All of the Baycrest Terrace subjects used Arabic numbers and placed them inside the contour. Analysis of the type of errors showed that some subjects in each of the LoDRS

TABLE 4-4.   Total Clock Score in Baycrest Terrace Subjects

	DRS < 123	DRS ≥ 123	*p*
Free-Drawn Clock			
(max=15)			
11:10			
Mean	9.5	13.2	*p* < 0.05*
SD	3.3	1.7	
N	6	19	
8:20			
Mean	11.0	13.1	NS
SD	2.5	1.8	
N	5	19	
3:00			
Mean	10.6	13.2	*p* < 0.05
SD	2.2	1.7	
N	5	19	
Examiner Clock			
(max=11)			
11:10			
Mean	6.0	9.6	*p* < 0.05
SD	3.8	1.5	
N	8	17	
8:20			
Mean	6.5	10.1	*p* < 0.05
SD	3.3	1.6	
N	8	17	
3:00			
Mean	7.6	10.1	*p* < 0.05
SD	3.0	0.7	
N	8	17	

* Two-tailed Wilcoxon test.

and HiDRS subgroups placed the numbers in the incorrect position. As expected, the poor spacing tended to be more marked in the LoDRS subjects (Figure 4-1A,B versus Figure 4-3C,D). As indicated above, however, poor spacing of numbers occurs with sufficient frequency in normals that the significance of this finding must take into consideration the degree of incorrect number position rather than simply the presence of this error.

In contrast, omission of numbers rarely occurs in normals and suggests the presence of early deterioration in cognitive function when seen in elderly individuals. This is supported by the observation that the only subject in the HiDRS subgroup who omitted numbers had a DRS score of 126, which is just above the cutoff for "dementia" (Figure 4-4A). Furthermore, the severity of number omission was more marked in the subjects in the LoDRS subgroup (Figure 4-4B). Number omission should, therefore, make an examiner suspicious of significant deficits in cognitive function.

Ordering of numbers counterclockwise (Figure 4-3A) and placing numbers out of

TABLE 4-5.   Free-Drawn Clocks

	Percentage of Subjects with a Given Response*					
	DRS < 123			DRS ≥ 123		
	11:10 (n=6)	8:20 (n=5)	3:00 (n=5)	11:10 (n=19)	8:20 (n=19)	3:00 (n=19)
Contour						
Attempted	100.0	100.0	100.0	100.0	100.0	100.0
Acceptable	100.0	100.0	100.0	100.0	100.0	100.0
Numbers						
Only numbers 1–12 present	66.7	80.0	80.0	94.7	94.7	94.7
Arabic number representation	100.0	100.0	100.0	100.0	100.0	100.0
Numbers in correct sequence	66.7	60.0	80.0	100.0	100.0	100.0
Numbers drawn without rotating paper	100.0	100.0	100.0	94.7	89.5	89.5
Numbers in correct position	33.3	40.0	20.0	57.9	47.4	47.4
Numbers inside contour	100.0	100.0	100.0	100.0	100.0	100.0
Hands						
Two hands present	16.7	60.0	40.0	73.7	73.7	84.2
Hour target number indicated	83.3	80.0	80.0	100.0	100.0	100.0
Minute target number indicated	50.0	60.0	20.0	94.7	100.0	89.5
Hands in correct proportion	100.0	100.0	50.0	66.7	71.4	43.8
	(n=1)	(n=2)	(n=2)	(n=15)	(n=14)	(n=16)
No superfluous markings	50.0	80.0	100.0	100.0	100.0	100.0
Hands relatively joined	100.0	66.7	100.0	100.0	100.0	100.0
	(n=1)	(n=3)	(n=2)	(n=14)	(n=14)	(n=16)
Center						
Center is present (drawn or inferred)	50.0	60.0	80.0	73.7	73.7	89.5

* Percentage based only on subjects in whom the item could be scored. The sample size is shown in parentheses when less than the original total.

sequence (Figure 4-4B) were seen only in the LoDRS subgroup. These errors suggest the presence of significant cognitive deficits. This conclusion is supported by the normative study, which suggests that sequencing errors are pathological and cannot be attributed to normal aging. In contrast, rotation of the paper was seen in approximately 10 percent of the subjects between ages 70–79 and 80–89 years, suggesting that this response is associated with aging and should not be considered pathological.

To summarize, abnormalities in number drawing that were seen in the Baycrest Terrace subjects include omission of numbers, poor number positioning, and incorrect sequencing. As expected, these abnormalities were more common in individuals with lower DRS scores.

HANDS

There were also subjects in both subgroups who failed to draw two hands. Analysis of the types of errors, however, showed a marked difference in performance between

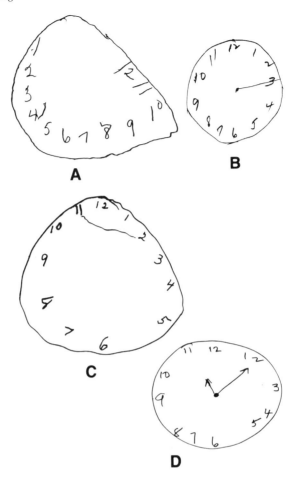

Figure 4–3   Range of good and poor contours. (A and B) LoDRS group; DRS 121, age 80 and DRS 112, age 87, respectively. (C and D) HiDRS group; DRS 132, age 80 and DRS 144, age 85, respectively. Also, the numbers in A are ordered counterclockwise.

subgroups. When the subjects in the HiDRS subgroup failed to place two hands on the clock, they either put a mark at the site of both target numbers (Figure 4-5A) or drew a line joining the minute and hour target numbers without demarcating two separate hands (Figure 4-5B). In the LoDRS subgroup, however, there were other types of responses that included drawing a curved line with a small arrowhead from the "10" to the "11" for "11:10" (Figure 4-1A), writing the number "10" on the clock face for "11:10" (Figure 4-1B), drawing a circular hand sweeping around inside the boundary of the clock face (Figure 4-2A), and drawing hands that point to incorrect numbers even though they are directed toward the appropriate location for "3 o'clock" on the clock face (Figure 4-4B). One subject in the HiDRS subgroup drew hands with arrows

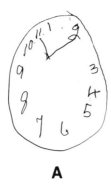

A

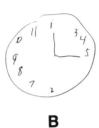

B

Figure 4–4   Examples of number omissions in patients with low normal DRS scores or scores below the cutoff of 123. (A) Omission of "12"; DRS 126, age 76. Note the upward pull of the center towards the target numbers. (B) Omission of "12" and "6"; DRS 113, age 79. The hands are drawn in the correct spatial position despite the incorrect target numbers. Also, the "2" is out of sequence.

on the ends pointing to the center in a reversed direction (Figure 4-5C). It is of interest that this subject's DRS score dropped 10 points from 132 into the "demented" range within 5 months of drawing the abnormal clock.

CENTER

Subjects in both the LoDRS and HiDRS subgroups did not always indicate a drawn or inferred center (i.e., if the nonconnected hands were extended they would not meet at a common point). Subjects in the LoDRS subgroup who had no center on their clocks, however, tended to draw very poor clocks in general (e.g., Figures 4-1B, 4-3A). In contrast, the lack of a center in many of the HiDRS subjects was essentially due to their poor representation of the hands such as drawing a straight line between the minute and hour target numbers (Figure 4-5B).

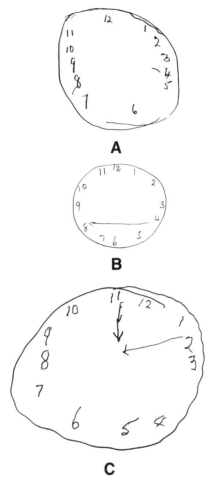

Figure 4–5   Examples of abnormal hands in the HiDRS group. (A) Marks at the site of the target numbers; DRS 129, age 75. (B) A line joining the two target numbers; DRS 137, age 88. (C) Arrows on the wrong end of the hands; DRS 132, age 89.

Examiner Clock Condition

Table 4-6 shows the quantitative performance profiles of the Baycrest Terrace subjects on each of the critical items for hands and center on the examiner clocks.

HANDS

All but one subject in the HiDRS subgroup drew two clearly demarcated hands that emanated from a drawn or inferred center on all three examiner clocks. The single subject who failed to draw two hands made this error on the "11:10" and "8:20" clocks

TABLE 4-6. Examiner Clocks

	Percentage of Subjects with a Given Response*					
	DRS < 123 (n=8)			DRS ≥ 123 (n=17)		
	11:10	8:20	3:00	11:10	8:20	3:00
Hands						
Two hands present	62.5	62.5	75.0	94.1	94.1	100.0
Hour target number indicated	87.5	100.0	100.0	100.0	100.0	100.0
Minute target number indicated	50.0	62.5	75.0	100.0	100.0	100.0
Hands in correct proportion	60.0	40.0	66.7	62.5	75.0	52.9
	(n=5)	(n=5)	(n=6)	(n=16)	(n=16)	
Hour hand/mark not displaced	85.7	87.5	62.5	93.8	100.0	87.5
	(n=7)			(n=16)	(n=16)	(n=16)
Minute hand/mark not displaced	66.7	83.3	66.7	100.0	100.0	100.0
	(n=6)	(n=6)	(n=6)	(n=16)	(n=16)	(n=16)
No superfluous markings	62.5	75.0	87.5	94.1	100.0	100.0
Hands relatively joined	80.0	100.0	100.0	100.0	100.0	100.0
	(n=5)	(n=5)	(n=6)	(n=16)	(n=16)	
Center						
Center is present (drawn or inferred)	62.5	62.5	75.0	94.1	94.1	100.0
Center is not displaced from the vertical axis	40.0	40.0	83.3	75.0	93.8	76.5
	(n=5)	(n=5)	(n=6)	(n=16)	(n=16)	
Center is not displaced from the horizontal axis	80.0	80.0	66.7	75.0	81.3	100.0
	(n=5)	(n=5)	(n=6)	(n=16)	(n=16)	

* Percentage based only on subjects in whom the item could be scored. The sample size is shown in parentheses when less than the original total.

but not on the "3:00" time setting (Figure 4-6). The error on the "11:10" and "8:20" clocks consisted of the subject drawing a single line between the hour and minute target numbers. It is of note that the "3:00" setting places less demands on the subjects because there is no requirement to recode the minute target number from one value to another.

An error analysis of the production of the subjects in the LoDRS subgroup who failed to draw two hands showed a different profile from that seen in the subjects in the HiDRS subgroup. The errors consisted of a mark beside the number "10" (Figure 4-7A), marks at the hour and minute target number (Figure 4-7B), and a line from the "12" to a point between the numbers "6" and "7" as well as a hand to the "3" (Figure 4-7C). One subject placed a "20" beside the "8" for "8:20" (Figure 4-7D). This represents a classical frontal response characterized by a very literal interpretation of "20" after "8." Another drew a "3" beside the "3" for "3:00" (Figure 4-7E).

All of the subjects except one individual in the LoDRS subgroup joined the hands that were drawn. Displacement of the hands appeared to be slightly more common in this subgroup, particularly in the case of the minute hand.

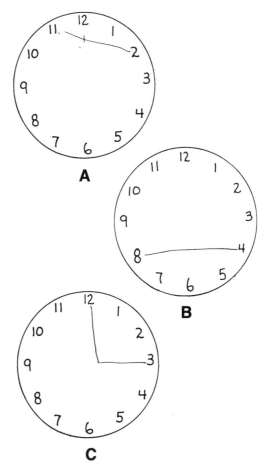

Figure 4–6   Examiner clocks showing differential sensitivity of the 11:10, 8:20, and 3:00 times for hands within a subject; DRS 137, age 88.

Superfluous marks were seen only in the LoDRS subgroup with the exception of one subject in the HiDRS subgroup who drew an extra hand on the "11:10" clock (Figure 4-2B). This subject, however, had one of the lowest DRS scores in the HiDRS subgroup (i.e., 126). Another example of a superfluous mark consisted of an extra hand on the "8:20" clock (Figure 4-8A).

CENTER

A center could be drawn or inferred in fewer subjects in the LoDRS subgroup as compared to the HiDRS subgroup. This reflected, however, the smaller number of subjects in the LoDRS subgroup who drew two hands. Table 4-7 shows the relationship

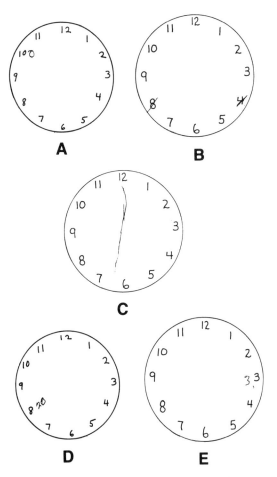

Figure 4–7 Examples on errors in drawing hands in the LoDRS group: (A) Mark at the hour target number; DRS 121, age 80. (B) Marks at the hour and minute target number; DRS 114, age 88. (C) A line between the 12 and the 6, as well as a hand to the 3; DRS 114, age 88. (D) a "20" beside the "8"; DRS 121, age 80. (E) a "3" beside the "3"; DRS 107, age 89.

between the time setting and the displacement of the center from the vertical and horizontal axes. Table 4-7 includes only those patients who had a significant displacement in either the horizontal direction (greater than 3.6 mm [¹/₈ in]) or vertical direction (greater than 5.1 mm [¹/₄ in] above or 3.6 mm below the horizontal axis). Although the numbers are small, the data suggest a tendency for the center to be displaced upwards for the "11:10" condition (Figure 4-4A). This may reflect a frontal pull to the upper half of the clock toward the "11" and "10." Similarly, for the "3:00" condition there seemed to be a pull to the right toward the "3" (Figure 4-6C). We also observed

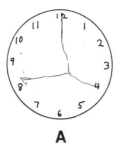

A

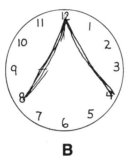

B

Figure 4–8   Abnormal hands in examiner clock condition. (A) An extra hand on the 8:20 clock; DRS 113, age 79. (B) Upward displacement of centre on 8:20 clock; DRS 139, age 84.

examples where the center was displaced to such an extent that the joining of the hands occurred at the number "12" (Figure 4-8B).

Comparing Times Set

We examined the relative sensitivity of the different time settings on both the free-drawn and examiner clocks in the Baycrest Terrace subjects. When setting the time to "10 after 11," "20 after 8," and "3 o'clock," subjects must recode the "10," "20," and the "o'clock" to a "2," "4," and "12," respectively, to represent correctly the minute hand. The subjects were more impaired on the free-drawn as compared to the examiner clocks. This is to be expected since there are no cues or structural elements available in the free-drawn condition to assist the subject.

Table 4-8 shows the relative frequency of a failure to indicate accurately the minute or hour hands in subjects who were able to draw two clock hands. Although errors occurred at each of the time settings, the type of incorrect response tended to differ. For the "11:10" setting, the errors included a stimulus-bound response, or frontal pull, to

TABLE 4-7. Relation Between Location of Center and Clock Time

	Left	Midline	Right	No. of subjects outside normal range
(a) 11:10 Setting				
Upper	3	3	1	7
Midline	0	—	0	0
Lower	1	0	2	3
Total	4	3	3	10
(b) 8:20 Setting				
Upper	0	0	3	3
Midline	0	—	1	1
Lower	1	1	1	3
Total	1	1	5	7
(c) 3:00 Setting				
Upper	0	0	1	1
Midline	1	—	1	2
Lower	0	1	2	3
Total	1	1	4	6

the "10" in two of the three incorrect free-drawn clocks and two of the four incorrect examiner clocks (e.g., Figure 4-2A).

For the "8:20" time setting, there was a failure to indicate the minute target number in two of the three incorrectly drawn free-drawn clocks and in the third a placement of a hand at the wrong number. In the examiner clocks there was one instance of a frontal response with a "20" placed after the "8" (Figure 4-7D). The other errors consisted of failure to indicate a target minute number or drawing a hand to the wrong target minute number.

For the "3:00" condition, the errors almost all consisted of a failure to indicate the "12" position for the minute hand (e.g., Figure 4-3B). Moreover, we observed that the "3:00" time setting may be relatively insensitive to bringing out abnormal responses compared to the "11:10" and "8:20" settings in some patients (Figure 4-9).

Therefore, in subjects with relatively mild cognitive impairment (i.e., residential elderly), all three clock times are sensitive for detecting impairment in setting the hands. Frontal responses appear to be more common for the "11:10" and "8:20" conditions, whereas omission of the minute hand appears to be the predominant error for the "3:00" condition.

Comparison of Clock-Drawing Task to Standard Measures

In the Baycrest Terrace subjects, the total clock score using the critical items from the normative scoring system was significantly correlated to performance on the DRS for

TABLE 4-8. No. of Subjects Failing to Indicate Minute or Hour Hand in Those Who Were Able to Draw Two Hands

Time Setting	Free-Drawn Clock	Examiner Clock	Total
11:10	3	4	7
8:20	3	3	6
3:00	6	2	8
Total	12	9	21

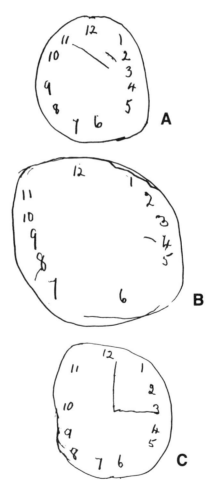

Figure 4–9   Free-drawn clocks show differential sensitivity of the 11:10, 8:20, and 3:00 times for hands within a subject; DRS 129, age 75.

all clock conditions ($r = .44, p < .05$). Based on the normative study in Chapter 2, we had established cutoff scores for performance on clock drawing. For the free-drawn clock, which was sensitive to deficits in the Terrace subjects in terms of the total clock score, there were no individuals among the Baycrest Terrace subjects with a score of 123 or more on the DRS, which is in the "nondemented" range, who fell below the cutoff. Impaired performance on clock drawing was, therefore, highly associated with "cognitive impairment."

In contrast to the relation with the DRS, performance on clock drawing was not significantly correlated to scores on the Raven's Coloured Progressive Matrices, a measure of nonverbal reasoning ability (Raven, 1965). The lack of significant correlation between this task and clock-drawing ability is consistent with the factor analysis described in the normative chapter, which showed a low correlation between clock-drawing ability and measures of general intellectual functioning, but a strong relationship between clock drawing and visual-analytic ability.

Conclusions

Clock drawing is a useful screening tool for assessing visual-analytic ability in the elderly living in a seniors' residence. Using the "critical items" scoring system described in the normative study (Chapter 2), statistically significant differences in the total clock scores were found between the subjects who were significantly impaired on the DRS as compared to those individuals with scores in the normal range. Although all subjects were able to draw an acceptable contour on the free-drawn condition, differences between the subgroups above and below the DRS cutoff for "dementia" were observed in the sequencing, omission, and positioning of the numbers, as well as in the drawing of the clock hands. On the examiner clocks, differences between the groups were noted in the drawing of the hands and displacement of the center.

A comparison between the three settings of "11:10," "8:20," and "3:00" showed them to be sensitive to the presence of cognitive deficits, but that the types of errors differed according to the time setting. Frontal types of responses were more prominent for the "11:10" and "8:20" clocks, whereas a failure to indicate the "12" position (i.e., an omission error), was most prominent on the "3:00" setting.

Quantitative comparison of the subjects living in the seniors' residence with a matched sample from the community showed that the total clock score on the free-drawn clock, but not on the examiner clock, was useful for discriminating between the two groups. Analysis of the performance scores on the critical items showed that the residential elderly differed from the normal controls essentially in their poor positioning of the numbers. This suggests that the ability to position numbers on a clock correctly may be one of the earliest clock-drawing changes to emerge as cognitive function declines in the elderly.

5. Focal Brain Damage

There have been few investigations of clock drawing as a diagnostic instrument, and those that are available have focused mainly on the elderly or on patients with neurodegenerative disorders that affect multiple brain regions. In an early study, Shulman and colleagues (1986) developed a limited scoring procedure for evaluating clock drawing and showed that performance on their version of the clock test correlated significantly with scores on two widely used tests of cognitive status, the Mini-Mental State Examination and the Short Mental Status Questionnaire. They also reported that clock drawing was adversely affected in patients with organic mental disorder and major affective disorder, and that impairment and improvement on clock drawing paralleled decline and recovery. Subsequently, other investigators found clock drawing to be sensitive to severity of dementia and a potentially useful test to screen for early Alzheimer's disease (Wolf-Klein et al., 1989; Sunderland et al., 1989; Tuokko et al., 1992).

Recently, Rouleau and co-workers (1992) used clock drawing to compare cognitive deficits associated with Alzheimer's disease and Huntington's disease. Both groups of patients produced abnormal drawings, but their respective impairments were qualitatively different. Patients with Alzheimer's disease made more perseverative errors and displayed rigid stimulus-bound behavior that reflected poor understanding and conceptualization of the task. Patients with Huntington's disease had difficulty managing graphic details, with frequent distortions of the clock face and poorly drawn numbers. In addition, the clocks drawn by subjects with Huntington's disease revealed sequencing and planning deficits that were attributed to damage within the frontal-striatal system.

The study by Rouleau and colleagues (1992) showed that clock drawing can be effectively used to distinguish between neurological conditions due to different pathology. Their results point to the potential value of clock drawing as a neuropsychological instrument for assessing functional impairments resulting from selective brain damage. Indeed, it has been noted that the visuospatial and planning demands of clock-drawing tests render them particularly sensitive to effects of lesions in the parietal lobe (Critchley, 1953) and frontal lobe (Albert & Kaplan, 1980).

In this chapter we describe clock drawing in patients with unilateral focal lesions. We shall first provide a clinical overview of the types of errors that occur after focal brain damage due to stroke by citing representative examples of the more typical focal lesion clocks seen by Drs. E. Kaplan and D. Delis over the years (Delis & Kaplan, 1983). We shall then present a formal analysis of clock drawing in a series of patients with focal brain lesions based upon the scoring system developed in the normative study. This formal analysis was carried out in a clinical population comprised primarily of patients with focal lesions due to tumor.

General Overview of Clock Drawing in Stroke Patients

LESIONS IN POSTERIOR AREAS OF THE RIGHT HEMISPHERE

One of the most pronounced sequelae of unilateral right posterior lesions is spatial disorganization (Benton, 1985b; Delis, Kiefner, & Fridlund, 1988; Kaplan, 1988). The clock drawings of these patients often contain all the essential elements (clock circle, numbers, and hands) but the features are scattered or distorted (Figure 5-1B). When elements are omitted, they tend to be the more nonverbal features (i.e., the hands and outer circle; Figure 5-1A,B), but not the verbal elements (i.e., the numbers). Left hemi-inattention (Heilman, Watson, & Valenstein, 1985), however, often results in omission of numbers on the left side of the clock (Figure 5-2B,C). Severe spatial

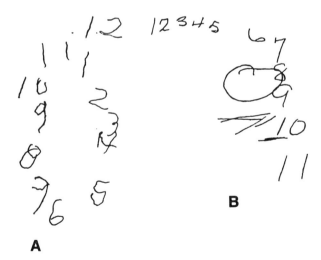

A   **B**

Figure 5–1   Clocks drawn by patients with large posterior lesions in the right hemisphere revealing (A) omission of outer configuration and hands; (B) severe spatial disorganization, left hemi-inattention, and a possible confusion of "12" as "1" and "2."

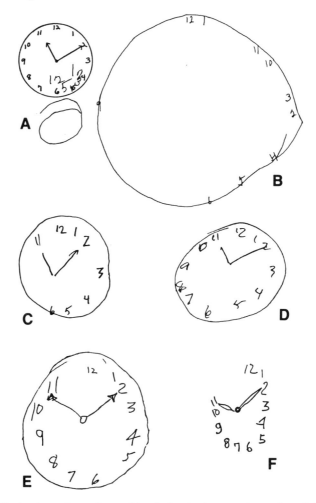

Figure 5–2   Clocks drawn by patients with a lesion in the posterior region of the right hemisphere, illustrating (A) spatial disorganization of numbers and omission of hands on copy task; (B) lesion in posterior right hemisphere showing spatial disorganization of numbers and left hemi-inattention; (C & D) lesion in right parietal lobe showing spatial disorganization (i.e., left neglect) on the copy version (C) but not on command (D); (E & F) right temporal lobe lesion illustrating more spatial disorganization (i.e., omission of outer configuration and inattention to spatial layout of number) on the command condition (F) than on copy condition (E).

disorganization may result in errors in sequencing numbers (Figure 5-2B). Even in copying a model clock, spatial disorganization is often salient (Figure 5-2A). The patient who drew the clock in Figure 5-2A became so disoriented after drawing a clock circle that he started to write the numbers within the model.

As noted above, the tasks of copying a clock and drawing a clock to oral-verbal command differentially tax cognitive functions. Copying places maximal demands on perceptual functions associated with the right parietal region. Accordingly, a lesion restricted to this area is more likely to impair performance on a copy condition relative to a command condition. For example, left inferior quadrant inattention was evident in a right parietal patient's clock to copy (Figure 5-2C) but not in his clock drawn to command (Figure 5-2D). In contrast, a command condition places maximal demands on memory and visual imagery, and thus damage to the temporal region is more likely to disrupt performance in this condition. Figure 5-2E,F illustrates a right temporal patient's errors of omission of the clock circle and poor planning in his command clock but not in his clock to copy. Dissociations in the performances of patients with right parietal and right temporal lobe lesions have been reported using other visuospatial tasks as well (Newcombe, Ratcliffe, & Damasio, 1987).

LESIONS IN ANTERIOR AREAS OF THE RIGHT HEMISPHERE

Patients with small right frontal lesions frequently show at least mild spatial impairment, especially in the command condition. Left hemi-inattention is usually absent, but there is sometimes a shift of the numbers on the left side toward the right (Figure 5-3A,B). Another spatial deficit is misorientation of arrow-hands (e.g., the minute hand in Figure 5-3B).

The frontal lobes play an essential role in integrating multiple dimensions of a task (Luria, 1980; Stuss & Benson, 1986). Consequently, patients with right frontal lesions are often unable to execute two aspects of a task simultaneously. In drawing a clock, the patient with a right frontal lesion often attends to only one parameter of the task (i.e., the predominantly left hemisphere function of generating the number sequence) and fails to maintain the correct spatial layout of the numbers simultaneously (Figure 5-3C). When a patient with unilateral right hemisphere damage leaves a gap at the end of the number sequence on the left side (Figure 5-3C), it is often unclear whether the error is due to impaired simultaneous processing (often associated with right anterior damage) or left hemi- inattention (often associated with right posterior damage).

Additional tasks may be used to test the examiner's hypotheses about the cognitive mechanisms that underlie this error. Asking the patient to draw the petals of a daisy may indicate whether or not he or she will draw them completely around the left hemispace, since there is no upper limit to the number of petals on a flower as there is to the numbers on a clock. The examiner can also determine whether the patient displays left hemi-inattention on other constructional tasks (e.g., WAIS-R NI Block Design subtest; Kaplan, Fein, Morris, & Delis, 1991).

Finally, it is important to note whether the patient shows awareness of his gap on the left side of the clock when he finishes writing the "11." If so, this would suggest that the patient was temporarily attending only to the one task of number writing, but that he did have the capacity to appreciate the incorrect spatial layout once he finished generating the numbers.

As noted above, the "10 after 11" clock often elicits the stimulus-bound response of setting the hands on "10" and "11" in patients with frontal lobe or diffuse pathology

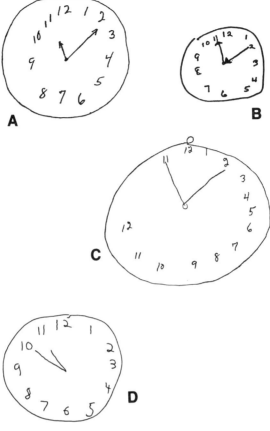

Figure 5–3   Clocks drawn by patients with focal lesions in frontal region of the right hemisphere, illustrating (A) shift of numbers on the left side to the right; (B) right-left, reversal of one hand; (C) attention to one parameter of the task—the sequencing of numbers—while not simultaneously maintaining the correct spatial layout of the numbers; (D) the stimulus-bound response of setting the hands on "10" and "11."

(Figure 5-3D). This deficit will appear only in a command condition since the hands are already set in a copy condition.

LESIONS IN POSTERIOR AREAS OF THE LEFT HEMISPHERE

Patients with lesions in the left temporoparietal region may have a Wernicke's aphasia (Goodglass & Kaplan, 1983), which compromises their understanding of the verbal instructions in the command condition. If language comprehension is severely impaired, the patient may not grasp the task set at all. In less severe cases of aphasia, the patient may understand the general task, but comprehension of the specific time setting may elude him or her. When a time setting is incorrect, hypothesis testing is needed to determine whether the error is related to aphasia or to a short-term memory problem. Results from additional language and memory testing will often clarify the underlying neurocognitive deficit. Aphasic patients will, of course, perform significantly better in the copy condition, because it places less demand on verbal comprehension.

Lesions in the left temporoparietal region may also result in agraphia. If the agraphia is mild, numbers can still be produced, but sequencing or rotation errors will occur. In severe agraphia, the numbers will be omitted in both command (Figure 5-4A) and copy (Figure 5-4D) conditions. Patients with severe agraphia may use the compensatory strategy of substituting some type of mark for the numbers (Figure 5-4B,C). Thus, whereas patients with right hemisphere damage are more likely to include the numbers than the more spatial features (i.e., clock circle and hands), patients with left hemisphere damage display the opposite pattern of performance. Patients with left-sided

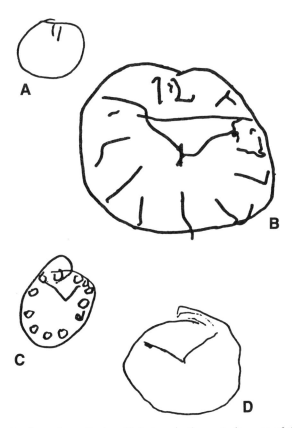

Figure 5–4   Clocks drawn by patients with lesions in the posterior area of the left hemisphere, illustrating (A) omission of the hands and numbers with the exception of one of the salient numbers, "11"; (B & C) compensation of numerical agraphia by drawing strokes or small circles in place of the numbers; (D) omission of numbers secondary to numerical agraphia on a copy task.

brain damage also rarely display right hemi-inattention (Heilman, Watson, & Valenstein, 1985).

Patients with left-posterior pathology sometimes set the hands on "10" and "11." The mechanism of this error could be related to impaired comprehension of the word "after" secondary to paragrammatism or stimulus-bound responding; thus, hypothesis testing is needed. A thorough evaluation of the nature and extent of a patient's language-comprehension skills will assist in making this differential diagnosis.

LESIONS IN ANTERIOR AREAS OF THE LEFT HEMISPHERE

The left frontal lobe has been implicated in the regulation and inhibition of verbal behavior (Luria, 1980). When a left frontal patient begins writing a number or line, he or she often has difficulty terminating the motor response, resulting in "overwriting" or motor persistence. Perseveration of numbers is another common manifestation of disinhibition in these patients.

Patients with left frontal lesions who have nonfluent aphasia often appear to have intact verbal comprehension; however, they often have a selective impairment in comprehending function words, such as prepositions, pronouns, and articles, with normal understanding of content words such as substantive nouns and verbs (Goodglass & Kaplan, 1983). Thus, when these patients are presented with a sentence that requires accurate processing of function words, such as the "after" in "10 after 11," they may set the hands at "10 *to* 11."

Patients with left hemisphere lesions tend to initiate constructional responses on the left side of the clock, that is, in the hemispace contralateral to their intact right hemisphere. As a result, they may write in the correct number sequence but in a counterclockwise direction, beginning with "12, 11, 10," etc. Occasionally, a patient with a left frontal lesion will not only write the numbers counterclockwise but will also reverse the sequence, resulting in a mirror reversal. Other spatial errors in writing that occur in these patients are up-down reversals (e.g., the "6" in Figure 5-5A) and right-left reversals (e.g., the "3" in Figure 5-5B).

Figure 5-6 displays clocks drawn by patients with global aphasia who had extensive damage in the distribution of the left middle cerebral artery. These clocks illustrate extreme forms of many of the deficits commonly found in patients with left-sided brain damage: reversed sequencing of numbers; agraphia; failure to comprehend the time setting (11:10); and omission of numbers.

Focal Brain Damage and Normative Scoring System

In the previous section we provided a clinical overview of the types of clocks that have been described after focal brain damage. In this section we demonstrate how the formal scoring system developed in the normative chapter can be applied to the quantitative analysis of clocks drawn by patients with focal lesions due primarily to tumor. The clock drawings of the patients were analyzed with an emphasis on the items designated

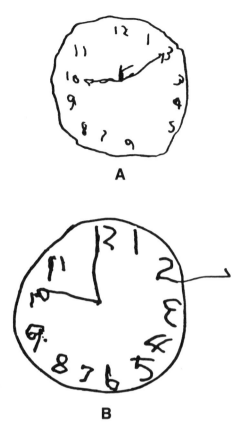

A

B

Figure 5–5 Clocks drawn by patients with large lesions in the anterior region of the left hemisphere, illustrating (A) perseveration of "3," and up-down reversal of the 6; (B) impaired comprehension of time setting, right-left reversal of "3."

as "critical" in the normative study. In addition, several other items from the initial 43-item scoring protocol (Appendix 2) were found to be especially useful in assessing cognitive disorders following brain damage. Deficits identified in the quantitative analyses are also described to clarify the nature of the respective impairments and the characteristic features of drawings associated with each type of lesion.

Where possible, free-drawn, pre-drawn, and examiner clocks were administered according to the procedures followed in the normative study and described in Chapter 2. In the free-drawn condition, subjects were given a blank sheet of paper and asked to draw a clock with all the numbers. They were then asked to set the clock at a specified time, usually "6:45," although occasionally other times (e.g., "8:20," "3 o'clock") were used. In the pre-drawn condition, subjects were presented with a circle drawn by the examiner and instructed to write in the numbers and to set the clock at a certain time, usually "6:05." In the examiner condition, subjects were given a circle in which

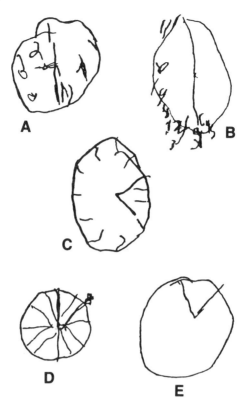

Figure 5–6   Clocks drawn by patients with global aphasia and extensive damage in the distribution of the left middle cerebral artery, illustrating (A) initiation of number sequencing on the left side, reversed sequencing of numbers, severe numerical agraphia after "3," more distortion of numbers written on the right side, and incorrect time setting; (B) initiation of number sequencing on the left side, severe numerical agraphia, and incorrect time setting; (C) numerical agraphia and incorrect time setting; (D) the "spoke" clock in which two hands were incorrectly set at two o'clock, followed by perseveration of hands; (E) omission of numbers secondary to agraphia.

the numbers on the clock were already drawn. They were asked to set the clocks at one or more of the following times: "8:20," "3 o'clock," "11:10."

Because many of the clocks were administered before standardized procedures were developed, considerable variation exists in the number and type of clocks administered to each patient. Moreover, several clocks were obtained from existing medical files and, occasionally, it was difficult to verify the precise procedures followed in administering those clocks. In all cases, however, information related to type of clock and time setting were available.

The majority of patients with frontal and parietal lesions had unilateral focal damage due to tumor (meningioma). Some patients, however, had suffered a stroke. Because the patients with meningiomas were seen after surgery, and because the tumors had compressed the brain from the external surface, we did not expect the deficits on clock drawing to be as severe as that described above after a stroke. The location and extent of damage was identified through case files, which often included a CT scan and, in the tumor cases, surgeons' reports. Patients with temporal lobe lesions had undergone temporal lobectomy as treatment for epilepsy. The clock drawings of each patient group were compared with those of age-matched normal control subjects who were tested as part of the normative study.

Analysis of Clock Drawings

Both quantitative and qualitative assessments were made of all clocks drawn by patients in the various groups. The initial quantitative analyses were based upon the critical items identified in the normative study (Chapter 2). Following the procedure of the normative study, a critical item score was obtained for each clock. Since not all the critical items were common to the various conditions, the maximal obtainable score for a given clock varied with the condition. To obtain an overall measure of clock-drawing ability, each patient's score was transformed to a percentage value and a mean percentage score was calculated for the group. The patient group means are presented in Table 5-1, along with the corresponding scores of the appropriate control groups.

Following examination of the entire set of clocks, we modified the original list of critical items to include items from the initial 43-item response protocol (Appendix 2) that appeared to be particularly sensitive to the differential effects of brain damage in our patients. The items that comprised this modified list assessed drawings of arrows (items 26, 27), hands (items 21, 22, 23), and displacement of hands from the center (items 35, 40, 36, 41, 38, 43). Tables 5-2 through 5-4 provide the average scores for the patient and control groups on these items as follows:

TABLE 5-1. Mean percentage scores for all groups based on critical items of the normative study.

Right Frontal	Left Frontal	Control
86.3	93.7	96.5
Right Parietal	Left Parietal	
93.1	70.0	96.5
Right Temporal	Left Temporal	
93.1	90.0	97.7

Note: Scores are expressed as a percentage of the maximum obtainable score.

**Item
No.**

Arrows

26	Both Hands	% clocks in which arrows were clearly drawn on both hands
27	Displacement	% clocks in which arrows were displaced from both hands by at least 1 mm ($^1/_{32}$ in)

Hands

21	Proportion	% clocks in which both hands were drawn in correct proportion to each other
22	Displacement	(Hour hand) $\overline{X}$ displacement in degrees of hour hand from target number
23	Displacement	(Minute hand) $\overline{X}$ displacement in degrees of minute hand from target number

Displacement of Center

35, 40	Vertical	$\overline{X}$ displacement in mm of drawn or inferred/extrapolated center from vertical axis
36, 41	Horizontal	$\overline{X}$ displacement in mm of drawn or inferred/extrapolated center from horizontal axis
38, 43	Center	$\overline{X}$ displacement in mm of drawn or inferred/extrapolated center from examiner's center

TABLE 5-2.   Frontal Lobe Damage

	Right Frontal	Left Frontal	Control
Hands (item no.)			
21 Proportion (% correct)	60.7	56.3	80.6
22 Displacement, hour hand (degrees)	10.7	2.5	4.5
23 Displacement, minute hand (degrees)	28.1	6.3	2.0
Arrows (item no.)			
26 Both Hands (% correct)	64.3	100.0	75.4
27 Displacement (% more than 1 mm)	82.6	12.5	36.4
Displacement of center (item no.)			
35, 40 Vertical axis (mm)	1.85	.88	.27
36, 41 Horizontal axis (mm)	4.0	.94	.76
38, 43 Examiner's center (mm)	4.96	2.13	2.45

Note: Scores for patients with right or left frontal lobe lesions and control group (aged 50–69 years) on items identified as being sensitive to effects of brain damage.

TABLE 5-3.　Parietal Lobe Damage

	Right Parietal	Left Parietal	Control
Hands (item no.)			
21 Proportion (% correct)	50.0	0.0	80.6
22 Displacement, hour hand (degrees)	0.0	28.6 (14)*	4.5
23 Displacement, minute hand (degrees)	6.2	62.5 (8)	2.0
Arrows (item no.)			
26 Both Hands (% correct)	73.3	50.0 (10)*	75.4
27 Displacement (% more than 1.0 mm)	0.0	100.0 (2)	36.4
Displacement of center (item no.)			
35, 40 Vertical axis (mm)	1.70	1.14	.27
36, 41 Horizontal axis (mm)	1.35	2.71	.76
38, 43 Examiner's Center (mm)	2.17	2.71	2.45

Note: Scores for patients with right or left parietal lobe damage and control group (aged 50–69 years).

* Some clocks could not be scored because of absent or poorly drawn hands or arrows. Numbers in parentheses denote the number of clocks out of 23 that were scored.

TABLE 5-4.　Temporal Lobe Damage

	Right Temporal	Left Temporal	Control
Hands (item no.)			
21 Proportion (% correct)	97.3	92.5	89.4
22 Displacement, hour hand (degrees)	2.7	2.5	5.5
23 Displacement, minute hand (degrees)	0.0	10.0	4.5
Arrows (item no.)			
26 Both hands (% correct)	100.0	95.0	72.1
27 Displacement (% more than 1 mm)	40.5	40.4	37.8
Displacement of center (item no.)			
35, 40 Vertical axis (mm)	.97	.93	.26
36, 41 Horizontal axis (mm)	1.65	1.19	.54
38, 43 Examiner's Center (mm)	2.24	1.70	2.48

Note: Scores for patients with right or left temporal lobe damage and control group (aged 20–39).

The clocks were also assessed qualitatively in an attempt to characterize features that may be associated with each type of focal brain lesion. This analysis enabled a process-oriented interpretation of the deficits revealed by the drawings. To support the qualitative analysis, typical examples of clocks for each group are provided and discussed.

As indicated in the previous section, clock drawings for the patient groups were made available through a variety of sources. As a result, there was considerable variation in the administration of the tests and the type of clocks that patients were asked to draw. In view of this, and because the numbers of patients in some groups were relatively small, it was not always possible to conduct a meaningful analysis of clocks in terms of type (free-drawn, pre-drawn, examiner) or time setting (e.g., "6:45," "8:20," "3 o'clock"). Consequently, scores for each item were collapsed across clocks into an overall score for each patient. To the extent that there were differences that could be related to specific features of clocks, they were assessed individually and are reported in the sections dealing with qualitative analysis.

Frontal Lobe Damage

The anterior portions of the frontal lobes mediate executive functions that are essential for organizing information and planning complex behavior. Damage to this region interferes with abstract thought processes necessary for the ability to develop appropriate strategies and hypotheses, to program movements, and to engage in divergent thinking. Typically, intellectual function, as measured by tests of general intelligence, is not affected in patients with frontal lobe damage. However, patients with frontal lobe damage are deficient in forming conceptual representations of a situation and, consequently, their behavior is characterized by highly concrete responses to specific stimuli. Patients consistently display a lack of spontaneity, faulty problem-solving and goal-directed behavior, and a rigidity that is frequently manifested by a tendency to perseverate on previously given responses (Luria, 1980; Stuss & Benson, 1986).

Although there are reports of memory disturbances in patients with prefrontal lesions, it is unlikely that such patients are deficient in forming a memory trace or in the straightforward recall of specific information. Their impairment on certain tests of memory probably reflect a retrieval deficit resulting from organizational difficulties that prevent a strategic search through memory (Moscovitch, 1989). Another aspect of memory that is impaired in frontal lobe patients is working memory, which some investigators have referred to as the process of integrating past experience with current events for the purpose of effective decision making (Moscovitch & Winocur, 1992).

Patients with frontal lobe lesions often show deficits in visuospatial function. As a result, they may be impaired on tests of spatial relations, especially those that require constructional abilities and the effective use of spatially distributed information. Semmes, Weinstein, Ghent, and Teuber (1963) compared the spatial deficits of patients with frontal or parietal lobe damage and concluded that they were qualitatively different. Patients with frontal damage were deficient mainly in orienting to objects in relation to their personal space, whereas patients with parietal lesions were impaired in forming relations between objects in extrapersonal space.

Clock-drawing tasks, because of their reliance on planning, attending to multiple stimulus parameters, and constructional abilities, should be highly sensitive to the effects of frontal lobe damage. Indeed, specific deficits on the clock test have been related to known or suspected lesions in areas of the frontal lobe (Albert & Kaplan, 1980). Abnormal responses attributed to frontal lobe dysfunction include conceptual failures, planning deficits, and perseveration.

An example of a conceptual deficit is when a patient sets the time at "10 *to* 11" after having been instructed to set it at "10 *after* 11." To follow the instruction correctly, the "10 after" must be recoded as the numeral "2." Patients with frontal lobe damage have difficulty with this process. Moreover, because the number "10" is located immediately adjacent to the "11," there is a tendency for such patients to be "pulled" to the "10" and to set one hand on the "10" and the other on the "11." This deficit, along with other abnormalities, were noted in our series of frontal lobe patients and are described in the following sections.

Clock Drawing by Patients with Frontal Lobe Damage

Ten patients with unilateral damage to the right frontal (RF) lobe and five with left frontal (LF) damage were included in the study. Their average age was 62 years (range, 49 to 71 years). Patients who underwent neuropsychological testing generally performed within the normal range on tests of intelligence (e.g., WAIS) and memory (Wechsler Memory Scale). On the other hand, these patients were impaired on the Wisconsin Card Sorting Test (WCST). Three patients with LF lesions had verbal fluency deficits as measured by word list generation for the letters "F," "A," and "S." This was consistent with the expected effects of their lesion. For purposes of comparison, subjects who comprised the 50- to 69-year-old age groups in the normative study served as age-matched controls for the frontal lobe groups.

RIGHT FRONTAL: QUANTITATIVE ANALYSIS

The total clock score for the RF group was determined using the critical items of the normative study (Table 5-1). It was slightly lower than the corresponding score of the age-matched control group. On the other hand, patients with RF damage were consistently impaired on those items identified as being particularly sensitive to effects of brain damage (Table 5-2). This deficit extended to all versions of the clock.

Patients with RF lesions showed a greater tendency for their clock hands to be out of proportion relative to controls. Also, the clock hands drawn by the patients were displaced in relation to the target numbers (Table 5-2). The arrow measures yielded a pattern that was not seen in any of the other groups. The RF and control groups drew arrows on the hands at about the same rate, but there was a clear difference in terms of displacement of the arrows from the hands. Whereas a displacement of more than 1 mm ($^1/_{32}$ in) (item 27) was seen only 36 percent of the time in controls, that amount of displacement occurred in 83 percent of RF clocks in which arrows were drawn.

Another example of the tendency of the RF group to displace from a target occurred when the real or inferred centers of the clock hands were examined in terms of their relation to the vertical and horizontal axes, as well as to the clocks' real centers. As can be seen in Table 5-2, patients with RF damage were severely impaired on these measures.

RIGHT FRONTAL: QUALITATIVE ANALYSIS

An examination of clocks drawn by the patients with RF lesions showed that they were impaired on positioning the numbers (Figure 5-7A). They also had some difficulty placing the numbers along the periphery of the pre-drawn clocks with a tendency for the numbers on the left to be shifted toward the right (i.e., toward the hemispace contralateral to the intact hemisphere). A mild form of this deficit is shown in Figure

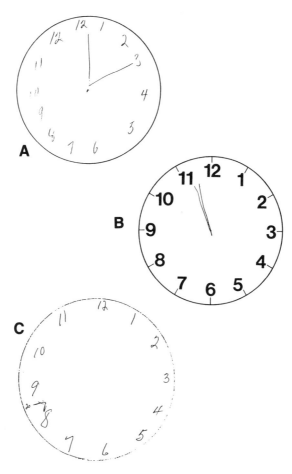

Figure 5–7   Clocks drawn by patients with right frontal lesions, illustrating (A) difficulty with number position; (B & C) stimulus-bound setting of hands.

5-7C). An example of a more severe deficit is shown in Figure 5-3A,B in the stroke patients. It should also be noted that the number "12" is repeated in the clock shown in Figure 5-7A. Although this response looks superficially perseverative, it more likely represents lack of attention to the "12" that had been drawn as the initial number. The likelihood is that the patient began with the number "12" at the top of the clock, as is usually the case, and then proceeded to draw the numbers from "1" to "12" without noticing that a "12" had already been placed on the clock face.

Patients with RF lesions were severely impaired at placing hands of the clocks in the correct positions (Figure 5-7B). Both hands were consistently drawn and usually joined, but they were typically in the wrong proportion (Figure 5-8B). The most frequent error of this type was to draw the hands the same length (Figure 5-8C). Of the various subject groups, the RF group had the most difficulty relating hour and minute hands to the center of the clock. As can be seen from Table 5-2, the real or inferred center of the hands was displaced an average of 4.96 mm ($^3/_{16}$ in); the average displace-

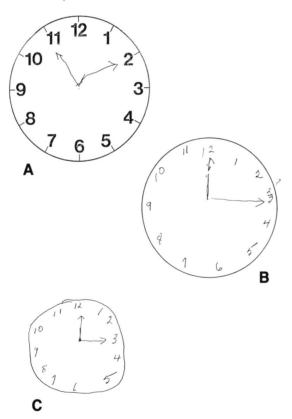

Figure 5–8   Clocks drawn by patients with right frontal lesions, illustrating (A) difficulty in drawing arrow on hands; (B) incorrect proportion of hands and number repetition; (C) incorrect proportion of hands and poor spacing of numbers.

ment for the other patient groups, which, for the most part, did not differ from each other (see Tables 5-3 and 5-4), was 2.19 mm ($^1/_{16}$ in). Similar deficits in the RF patients were seen along the vertical and horizontal axes. On some of the pre-drawn and examiner clocks, we attempted to help patients relate to the center of the clocks by providing a salient dot as a central reference point. This cue did not help the RF patients.

Patients with RF damage also made displacement errors when drawing hands in relation to the correct numbers (items 22, 23). This error was especially common for the minute hand, which was displaced an average of almost 30°. This was particularly apparent when the subject was required to recode the "10" in "11:10" or the "20" in "8:20." In Figure 5-7B, a line is drawn to a point just after the "11," and in Figure 5-7C the "20" is drawn in a very concrete representation.

Another displacement error that was reliably associated with RF damage occurred when patients attempted to draw arrows on minute and hour hands (item 27). The RF patients included the arrows about two-thirds of the time but, in over 80 percent of the attempts, the arrows were poorly drawn and displaced from the hands (see Figure 5-8A). Displacement errors appear to be a sensitive measure of RF damage and are probably a manifestation of the visuospatial deficits in such patients.

In summary, the planning, abstracting, and spatial orientation difficulties of patients with RF lesions are readily demonstrated by clock drawing. In general, their clocks contain all the essential elements but lack organization. The hands are invariably off-center and are usually displaced with respect to the correct numbers. When it is necessary to recode numbers, as in "11:10" or "8:20," there is a tendency to respond in terms of concrete stimulus features. The stimulus-bound nature of the deficit following RF lesions is also reflected in a tendency to repeat markings and overdraw concrete features of the clock. Although right-left reversals have been described in patients with anterior right hemisphere lesions due to stroke (Figure 5-3B), we did not observe this type of error in the sample of patients comprised primarily of postoperative tumor patients who were studied with the formal scoring system.

LEFT FRONTAL: QUANTITATIVE ANALYSIS

Patients with left frontal (LF) lesions did not differ from controls on the critical items of the normative study (Table 5-1). In general, their clocks were well drawn except for some difficulty in drawing the correct proportion of the hour and minute hands and an occasional tendency to include irrelevant markings. The LF subjects performed much better than did patients with RF damage on those items that assessed the effects of focal brain lesions (Table 5-2).

There was some indication that patients with LF damage had spatial difficulties with respect to drawing hands in the correct proportion (Figure 5-9C, D). Table 5-2 shows that in 56.3 percent of LF clocks the minute and hour hands were drawn in correct proportion whereas the corresponding number for age-matched controls was 80.6 percent.

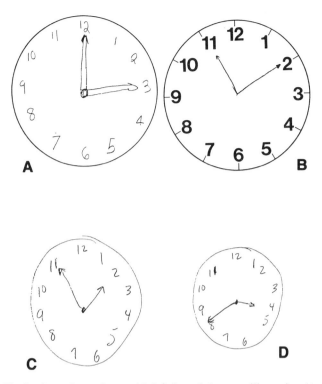

Figure 5–9   Clocks drawn by patients with left frontal damage, illustrating (A & B) normal minute hand placement; (C & D) reversal of the minute and hour hand proportion.

LEFT FRONTAL: QUALITATIVE ANALYSIS

The overall performance of patients with LF damage revealed some spatial difficulties, but the deficit was relatively mild and far less severe than that reliably produced by unilateral RF lesions. The LF patients drew better hands than did patients with RF damage although, as indicated above, they were not much better at drawing hands in the correct proportions. The LF patients produced fewer and less severe displacements of the hands than did the RF group. There was no indication of a frontal pull of the minute hand on either the "11:10" or "8:20" clocks (Figure 5-9B) in our limited sample. On the other hand, there was evidence of a tendency to reverse the length of the two hands.

There was an interesting finding with respect to arrow drawing (item 27). Whereas patients with RF lesions had a strong tendency to displace arrows from the minute and hour hands, patients with LF lesions drew well-formed arrows that invariably were in direct contact with the clock hands. Indeed, if anything, the patients with LF lesions performed better on this measure than did the control group (see Table 5-2).

In summary, while there were some signs of spatial and organizational deficits in clocks drawn by patients with LF damage, they were most pronounced in reproducing the relative proportion of the hands on the free-drawn clocks. These problems were much less apparent in the more structured pre-drawn and examiner clocks, confirming that the spatial disorientation produced by LF lesions was not as severe as that following RF lesions. In our sample, comprised primarily of postoperative surgical cases, we did not observe many of the abnormalities generally attributable to left anterior brain damage following stroke. These include initiating the number sequence on the left side—that is, contralateral to the intact right hemisphere—and thus writing the numbers in a counterclockwise sequence; mirror reversal of the numbers; up-down and left-right reversals (Figure 5-5A,B); and setting the hands at "10 to 11" for "10 after 11."

Parietal Lobe Damage

The postcentral gyrus in the anterior portion of the parietal lobe is the primary projection area for the somesthetic sensory system. Not surprisingly, damage to this region produces tactile sensory and perceptual deficits. In more posterior regions, input from several modalities provides the basis for a complex integrative function in which information from different sources is assimilated. This input converges mainly at the junction of the temporal, parietal, and occipital lobes in the angular gyrus, and damage here interferes with the ability to compare related information from different modalities.

Behavioral disturbances resulting from posterior damage have a decidedly spatial component. The spatial impairments of patients with parietal lesions have been described by numerous authors (e.g., Kaplan, 1988; Kolb & Whishaw, 1990; Lezak, 1983; Luria, 1981; Walsh, 1987) and include deficits in localizing and remembering stimuli in space and in forming topographical relationships between spatially distributed objects. Constructional impairment has also been reported in patients with parietal lesions, although there is disagreement as to whether this constitutes a separate entity. Some observers believe that constructional disabilities are related to deficits in spatial orientation or a disorder of body schema.

Unilateral parietal damage frequently produces deficits in attending to stimuli in space. Lesions in the right parietal lobe often produce a dramatic unilateral spatial neglect in which patients are unaware of objects on the left side. This deficit has been studied most extensively in the visual domain, but it also occurs in the auditory and tactile modalities. A particularly interesting attentional disorder associated with right parietal damage involves the recognition of well-known objects. Such patients are usually able to identify objects when they are drawn in a familiar way but not when they are presented in an unusual orientation. This deficit, first described by Warrington and Rabin (1970), has been viewed by some authors (e.g., Kolb & Whishaw, 1990)as another expression of spatial processing failure in patients with parietal damage.

Contralateral neglect is reported less frequently following lesions in the left parietal lobe. Lesions on the left side do, however, produce spatial deficits, such as right-left discrimination and difficulty processing internal details of figures. Left parietal damage also produces such disorders as aphasia, agraphia, alexia, acalculia (i.e., disorders that reflect an impaired use of language or symbols), and the Gerstmann syndrome (Gerstmann, 1940), which includes right-left disorientation, finger agnosia, agraphia, and acalculia.

The spatial nature of clock drawing suggests that this test should be sensitive to effects of parietal damage. Indeed, there are reports that patients with parietal lesions draw impoverished clocks that lack coherence and in which important elements are frequently missing. An important question to address is whether the spatially disorganized clocks of patients with parietal damage are similar to those of patients with frontal lobe lesions. If, as is widely assumed, the two types of lesion produce different spatial disorders, a comparison of clocks drawn by patients with parietal or frontal lobe lesions should yield distinguishable functional deficits.

Clock Drawing by Patients with Parietal Lobe Damage

Four patients with right parietal (RP) lesions and five with left parietal (LP) lesions were tested. Their average age was 66 years (range, 55–72 years). The most conspicuous feature of the neuropsychological data available for this group was a pronounced deficit on the Block Design subtest of the WAIS. Their performance was normal on tests of delayed recall and recognition and the Boston Naming Test. The control group for the parietal lobe patients was the 50- to 69-year-old subjects from the normative study.

RIGHT PARIETAL: QUANTITATIVE ANALYSIS

The patients with right parietal lobe damage did not differ from their age-matched controls on the critical items used in the normative study (Table 5-1). For the most part, the RP group also scored well on items found to be useful in differentiating clock drawings of the lesion groups (Table 5-3), although there were some signs of impairment.

The quantitative analysis showed that an area in which patients with RP lesions had difficulty was in drawing hands. As can be seen in Table 5-3, they displayed an impairment in drawing them in the right proportion (item 21). Moreover, the patients with RP lesions showed abnormal displacement of the center on the vertical (items 35, 40) and horizontal (items 36, 41) axes, although they did not differ from controls on center displacement. This pattern contrasts with that of the RF patients who displaced abnormally on all three measures.

RIGHT PARIETAL: QUALITATIVE ANALYSIS

Patients with RP lesions drew only three free-drawn clocks (two were drawn by the same patient) and they are presented in Figure 5-10. While deficient in several respects, the free-drawn clocks were more intact than might be expected on the basis of other reports of clock drawing by patients with RP damage (Albert & Kaplan, 1980).

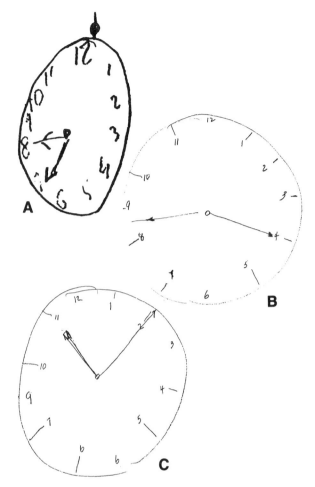

Figure 5–10   Clocks drawn by patients with right parietal lobe damage, illustrating (A) contour distortion; (B) hour hand displaced toward target number; (C) number repetition.

This most likely reflects the fact that our sample consisted primarily of postoperative patients who had meningiomas removed. The contours were somewhat distorted, (Figure 5-10A) but acceptable for presence of contour. The numbers were reasonably well oriented although not consistently well positioned in relation to each other. The numbers in Figure 5-10B,C were slightly removed from the periphery, but, in a sense, they were related to the outside of the circle by connecting lines.

There were signs of spatial disorientation involving the hands of free-drawn clocks. In Figure 5-10A, the hands are joined but off-center. The instruction for that clock was to set the hands at "6:45." The patient set the hands at the correct position but in the wrong proportion and at the incorrect target numbers. The hands on the "8:20" clock

(Figure 5-10B) are centered appropriately but they are drawn approximately the same length and are not joined in the center. Of note is that the hour hand is displaced, or pulled, away from the center toward the "8" in a stimulus-bound fashion. In Figure 5-10C the subject also drew an extra "6." It is likely that this is secondary to his having first placed the "12," "3," "6," and "9" as anchors to act as reference points, and when writing the automatized sequence of numbers he produced another "6." It is noteworthy that this error, as well as the omission of the "8" (Figure 5-10C), both occur on the left side of the clock.

Of the four pre-drawn clocks in our sample, three were well drawn. A typical good pre-drawn clock is shown in Figure 5-11A. One pre-drawn clock was poorly drawn (Figure 5-11B) and revealed a severe spatial problem in the placement of the numbers. As can be seen, the numbers showed poor positioning and spacing. Unusually large gaps can be noted between the "5" and "6" and between the "11" and "12," suggesting poor ability to plan the distribution of number placement. The center was displaced from the vertical axis, and the hands, which correctly indicated the time, were not joined. In the "3 o'clock" and "11:10" examiner clocks shown in Figures 5-11C,D, the

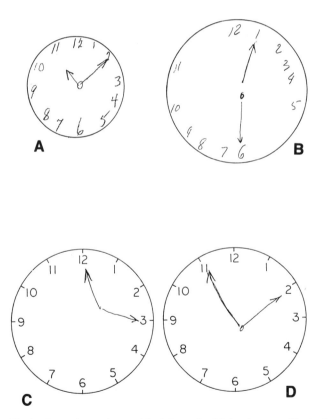

Figure 5–11   Clocks drawn by patients with right parietal lobe damage, illustrating (A) a good pre-drawn clock; (B) spatial deficit in number placement; (C & D) center displacement.

hour hands are virtually touching the "3" and "11," respectively, and the center in the "3 o'clock" drawing is significantly displaced toward the "3." These maybe considered signs of pulling to the more concrete number associated with the hour. Another feature of the examiner clocks drawn by RP patients is that the minute and hour hands were not well proportioned in relation to each other.

A notable feature of clocks drawn by RP patients was the absence of any evidence of contralateral neglect, as described in the general overview above and shown in Figure 5-2C. Also, while there were clear signs of spatial disorientation, the clocks did not suffer the lack of organization that has been described after stroke (see Figure 5-1B).

LEFT PARIETAL: QUANTITATIVE ANALYSIS

Quantitative analyses revealed severe impairments in the clocks drawn by patients with left parietal (LP) lesions. Their overall average score, based on critical items identified in the normative study, was 70.0 percent, as compared to 96.5 percent for age-matched control subjects (Table 5-1). On the critical items for brain-damaged patients, the patients with LP lesions were impaired on virtually every measure (Table 5-3).

The deficit was even greater than would appear from the scores indicated in Table 5-3 because of the patients' widespread failure to include essential features of the clocks. This was especially true with respect to items related to hand drawing. Of the 24 clocks drawn by patients with LP damage, only 13 included hands and, in only 8 of those, were two hands drawn. Since scores are expressed as percentages, based on total identifiable responses, measures referring to aspects of hand drawing (e.g., arrows, displacement from center) exclude several clocks in which two hands did not appear.

LEFT PARIETAL: QUALITATIVE ANALYSIS

The clocks produced by the LP subjects were of poor quality in all three drawing conditions. Figure 5-12A–D provides examples of free-drawn clocks that illustrate the lack of organization and perseveration characterizing clocks in this category. The clocks consistently reveal signs of poor drawing ability and impaired use of numbers, both of which are identified with LP lesions.

The clocks in Figure 5-12B,C show two attempts by one patient to draw numbers and represent "3 o'clock." The same patient could encode only the hour in trying to represent "11:10" and "8:20" on the examiner clocks (Figure 5-12E,F). Superficially, the two sets of drawings seem to reveal signs of neglect of the right side of space. However, spatial neglect is not common in patients with LP lesions, and a more plausible explanation is that the drawings reveal planning and recoding deficits. The extraneous markings outside the clocks, which were probably intended to help the patient attend to salient features of the clocks, may also reflect frontal lobe damage.

One patient showed strong perseverative tendencies by repeating numbers in a poorly organized free-drawn clock (Figure 5-12D). This pattern is more typical of frontal lobe damage, and there is further evidence that the lesion may have extended to frontal regions.

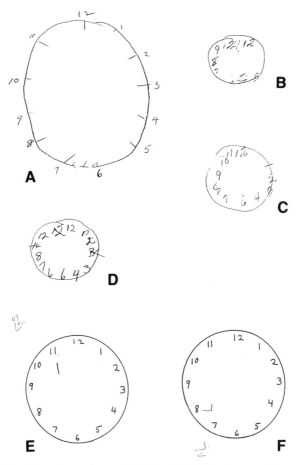

Figure 5–12   Clocks drawn by patients with left parietal lobe damage, illustrating (A-F) poor organization, number repetition, omission of hands, and extraneous markings.

As previously indicated, the LP patients had severely impaired pre-drawn and examiner clocks. In general, their pre-drawn clocks reveal poor organization and an inability to recode numbers. The recoding failure, shown in Figure 5-13A, was seen in two patients. Further evidence of the inability of the LP patients to draw correct times and their recoding problems is provided in their examiner clocks. In Figure 5-13B,C, this deficit is reflected clearly in clocks drawn by an LP patient. The instructions were to indicate "11:10" and "8:20," respectively, on the examiner clocks, but the actual times drawn were markedly incorrect.

When hands were present in the clocks, they were invariably drawn in the wrong proportion and consistently failed to indicate the correct times. When both hands were drawn (about 50 percent of the time), they were usually joined but displaced from the

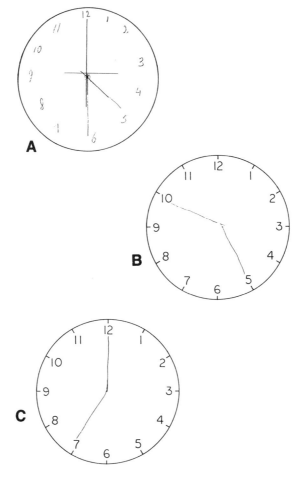

Figure 5–13   Clocks drawn by patients with left parietal lobe damage, illustrating recoding difficulty.

numbers associated with the correct times. As can be seen from Table 5-3, the latter score was worse for the LP group than the RP group. Interestingly, the displacement of the center of the clocks (mean = 2.71 mm) in the LP group was not unusually high for brain-damaged patients and substantially less than that of the RF group (mean = 4.96 mm). As for arrow-displacement, patients with LP damage drew so few arrows that no judgment could be made on this measure.

   In summary, LP damage severely impaired all aspects of clock drawing. The drawings reflected deficits in attending to spatial features, encoding the times, and in constructing the various elements. While some features of their clocks were reminiscent of frontal signs, the clocks drawn by the LP group were worse in almost all respects than those produced by patients with frontal lobe damage.

Temporal Lobe Damage

The temporal lobes are reliably identified with learning and memory functions. The classic work of Brenda Milner and her colleagues, involving patients with surgical excisions of temporal lobe structures, showed that lesions affecting the hippocampal region of the medial temporal lobe produce profound memory disturbances in all modalities. In patients with bitemporal damage, the most conspicuous feature is an anterograde amnesia in which the ability to recall new experiences is virtually obliterated. There is also evidence of a temporally graded retrograde amnesia in which the memory for older events is better than memory for events that occurred closer to the onset of damage. When damage is limited to the left hippocampus, memory loss may be restricted to verbal information, whereas selective hippocampal damage in the right hemisphere often produces memory loss primarily for nonverbal material (Milner, 1958, 1966).

Nonauditory perceptual disturbances, particularly in the visual modality, have also been reported in patients with temporal lobe lesions (Milner, 1958). These are undoubtedly the result of lesions affecting connections with posterior brain regions. Other effects of temporal lobe damage include hallucinations and disturbances of affect. The latter have been noted most frequently in patients suffering from temporal lobe epilepsy (Pincus & Tucker, 1974).

Our temporal lobe group includes patients with damage to left or right hemispheres. All displayed memory loss that was appropriate for the hemisphere involved, but there was no indication that other sensory, perceptual, or affective functions were disturbed. For the most part, the temporal lobe subjects drew very good clocks. Clock drawing requires that the patient make use of a general knowledge of clocks and their organization. This type of memory, namely semantic memory, does not depend on recall of specific experiences and is usually spared in temporal lobe amnesia. While patients must remember specific instructions pertaining to the task, the intervals involved are so brief as not to be affected by the memory disturbance. Thus, one might not expect a deficit in clock drawing arising from fundamental disturbances caused by temporal lobe damage.

Clock Drawings by Temporal Lobe Patients

Twelve patients with lesions to the left temporal (LT) lobe and eight with lesions to the right temporal (RT) lobe were tested. Their average age was 31 years (range, 23–41 years). Performance on a range of neuropsychological tests was generally normal. The only exception appears to have been with respect to memory function where all three of the LT patients tested on the Wechsler Memory Scale (Wechsler, 1945) (WMS) performed below normal. In contrast, all four patients with RT lesions, who were administered the WMS, scored at least within the normal range.

The 20- to 39-year-old subjects in the normative study served as age-matched controls for patients with temporal lobe lesions.

RIGHT TEMPORAL: QUANTITATIVE ANALYSIS

The average score for the RT group on the critical items of the normative study was similar to that of its age-matched control group (Table 5-1). The two groups were also very similar on those items used to assess brain damage (Table 5-4). The only area where RT patients did not do as well as controls was with respect to displacement of the drawn center along the vertical (items 35, 40) and horizontal (items 36, 41) axes in the free-drawn and pre-drawn clocks.

It is noteworthy that the RT patients drew the minute and hour hands in better proportion than any other patient group. Furthermore, all the RT patients drew arrows on both hands, and, in contrast to patients with RF lesions, they showed no evidence of displacing arrows from the hands.

RIGHT TEMPORAL: QUALITATIVE ANALYSIS

The clocks drawn by the RT patients in the free-drawn condition were generally of good quality. The contours were well formed, all the numbers were present in the correct orientation and position, and the hands accurately identified the time. However, these patients frequently mildly displaced the hands from the vertical and horizontal axes. A typical free-drawn clock drawn by RT patients is provided in Figure 5-14A,B.

The pre-drawn clocks yielded essentially the same pattern for numbers and hands. The numbers were reasonably well positioned, and the hands, for the most part, were in the correct proportions. Clocks drawn in the examiner condition were similarly remarkable (Figure 5-14C).

Delis and Kaplan (1983) noted a tendency toward heightened attention in temporal lobe epileptics that is manifested in unusual attention to detail and well-articulated clocks (Delis & Kaplan, 1983). One of our RT subjects drew a very similar clock, suggesting that, to the extent that this is a feature of temporal lobe dysfunction, it may be localized in the right hemisphere.

In summary, the clocks drawn by patients with RT damage scarcely differed from those drawn by normal age-matched control subjects. It should be emphasized, however, that more posterior lesions than those produced by temporal lobectomy may have resulted in more severe deficits.

LEFT TEMPORAL: QUANTITATIVE ANALYSIS

Quantitative analyses of the clocks drawn by patients with LT damage yielded essentially the same pattern of results as seen in the RT group (see Tables 5-1 and 5-4). The parallels even extended to superior performance, relative to controls, on the orientation, position, and spacing of the numbers. The one area where the RT and LT subjects may have differed was in displacement of the drawn center from the center as determined by the experimenter (items 38, 43). On this item, the LT subjects were slightly superior. While this result may point to a hemispheric effect, an unequivocal conclu-

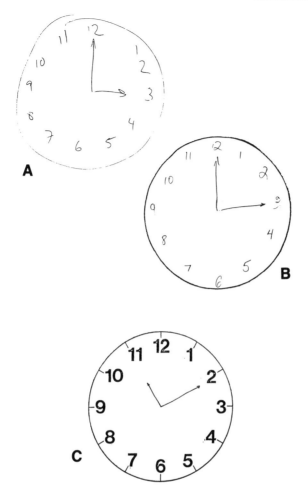

Figure 5–14 Clocks drawn by patients with right temporal lobe damage, illustrating (A) slight displacement of hands from vertical and horizontal axes; (B) failure to join hands at center; (C) well-drawn clock in examiner condition.

sion is clouded by the fact that the LT patients also outperformed the controls on the center-displacement measure.

LEFT TEMPORAL: QUALITATIVE ANALYSIS

As was the case with clocks drawn by the RT patients, patients with LT damage drew very good clocks that, for the most part, could not be differentiated from those drawn by controls. Examples of typical free-drawn, pre-drawn, and examiner clocks of patients with LT lesions are provided in Figure 5-15. There was, however, relatively

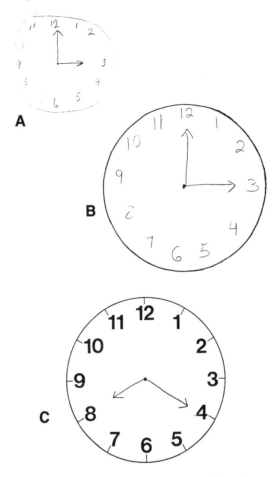

Figure 5–15   Clocks drawn by patients with left temporal lobe damage, illustrating typical (A) free-drawn; (B) pre-drawn; and (C) examiner clocks.

large displacement of the joined hands from the vertical and horizontal axes. This type of deficit was not specific to any single group. As for the right temporal lobe patients, we cannot rule out the possibility that more posterior lesions might have resulted in more severe deficits.

Summary and Conclusions

The data from this study using the scoring system developed in the normative study, as well as the findings based upon clinical experience, show that clock drawing can help differentiate the behavioural effects of focal brain damage. Moreover, clock drawing may also reveal different deficit profiles depending upon the type of brain pathology.

This was well illustrated by the differences in the clocks drawn by the patients with stroke as compared to those drawn by the patients with tumor.

Clock drawing is especially well suited to identify deficits in planning, abstraction, organizational, graphomotor, and spatial abilities associated with focal brain damage. A careful analysis of the strategies and errors that patients display in drawing clocks provides a valuable window into brain function and dysfunction. As such, the clock-drawing task often generates initial diagnostic hypotheses that can be tested using a comprehensive neuropsychological evaluation.

References

Adams, R. D., & Victor, M. (Eds.). (1989). *Principles of neurology* (4th ed.) (pp. 937–940). New York: McGraw-Hill.

Albert, M. S., & Kaplan, E. (1980). Organic implications of neuropsychological deficits in the elderly. In L. W. Poon, J. L. Fozard, L. S. Cermak, D. Arenberg, & L. W. Thompson (Eds.), *New directions in memory and aging.* Hillsdale. N.J.: Erlbaum.

Albert, M. S., & Moss, M. (1984). Assessment of memory disorders in patients with Alzheimer disease. In L. R. Squire & N. Butters (Eds.), *Neuropsychology of memory.* New York: The Guilford Press.

Andrews, K., Brocklehurst, J. C., Richads, B., & Laycock, P. J. (1980). The prognostic value of picture drawings by stroke patients. *Rheumatology and Rehabilitation, 19,* 180–181.

Battersby, W. S., Bender, M. B., Pollack, M., & Kahn, R. L. (1956). Unilateral "spatial agnosia" ("inattention") in patients with cortical lesions. *Brain, 79,* 68–93.

Benton, A. L. (1985a). Spatial thinking in neurological patients: Historical aspects. In L. Costa & O. Spreen (Eds.), *Studies in neuropsychology.* New York: Oxford University Press.

Benton, A. L. (1985b). Visuoperceptual, visuospatial, and visuoconstructional disorders. In K. M. Heilman & E. Valenstein (Eds.), *Clinical neuropsychology.* New York: Oxford University Press.

Benton, A. L., & des Hamsher, K. (1989). *Multilingual aphasia examination: Manual of instructions.* Iowa City, Iowa: AJA Associates.

Bowen, F. P., Kamienny, R. S., Burns, M. M., & Yahr, M. D. (1975). Parkinsonism: Effects of levodopa treatment on concept formation. *Neurology, 25,* 701–704.

Brun, A., & Englund, E. (1981). Regional pattern of degeneration in Alzheimer's disease. Neuronal loss and histopathological grading. *Histopathology, 5,* 549–564.

Butters, N., & Cermak, L. S. (1980). *Alcoholic Korsakoff syndrome: An information processing approach.* New York: Academic Press.

Chase, T. N., Foster, N. L., Fedio, P., et al. (1984). Regional cortical dysfunction in Alzheimer's disease as determined by positron emission tomography. *Annals of Neurology, 15*(Suppl.), S170–S174.

Coblentz, J. M., Mattis, S., Zingesser, L. H., Kasoff, S. S., Wisniewski, H. M., & Katzman, R. (1973). Presenile dementia: Clinical aspects and evaluation of cerebrospinal fluid dynamics. *Archives of Neurology, 29,* 299–308.

Cools, A. R., Van Der Bercken, J.H.L., Horstink, M.W.T., Van Spaendonck, K.P.M., & Berger, H.J.C. (1984). Cognitive and motor shifting aptitude disorder in Parkinson's disease. *Journal of Neurology, Neurosurgery and Psychiatry, 47,* 443–453.

Critchley, M. (1953). *The parietal lobes.* New York: Hafner Press.

Cummings, J. L., & Benson, D. F. (1983). *Dementia: A clinical approach.* Boston: Butterworths.

Cutler, N. R., Haxby, J. V., Duara, R., et al. (1985). Brain metabolism as measured with positron emission tomography: Serial assessment in a patient with familiar Alzheimer's disease. *Neurology, 35,* 1556–1561.

Dastoor, D. P., Schwartz, G., & Kurzman, D. (1991). Clock-drawing—An assessment technique in dementia. *Journal of Clinical and Experimental Gerontology, 13,* 69–85.

Delis, D. C., Direnfeld, L., Alexander, M. P., & Kaplan, E. (1982). Cognitive fluctuations associated with "on-off" phenomenon in Parkinson disease. *Neurology, 3,* 1049–1052.

Delis, D. C., & Kaplan, E. (1983). *The neuropsychology of "10 after 11."* Paper presented at the meetings of the International Neuropsychological Society, Mexico City.

Delis, D. C., Kiefner, M., & Fridland, J. A. (1988). Visuospatial dysfunction following unilateral brain damage: Dissociations in hierarchical and hemispatial analysis. *Journal of Clinical and Experimental Neuropsychology, 10,* 421–431.

Eddy, J. E., & Sriram, S. (1977). Clock-drawing and telling time as diagnostic aids. *Neurology, 27,* 595.

Flowers, K. A. (1982). Frontal lobe signs as a component of Parkinsonism. *Neurobehavioral Brain Research, 5,* 100–101.

Flowers, K. A., & Robertson, C. (1985). The effects of Parkinson's disease on the ability to maintain a mental set. *Journal of Neurology, Neurosurgery and Psychiatry, 48,* 517–529.

Folstein, M. F., Folstein, S. E., & McHugh, P. R. (1975). Mini-mental state: A practical guide for grading the cognitive state of patients for the clinician. *Journal of Psychiatric Research, 12,* 189–198.

Freedman, M., & Oscar-Berman, M. (1986). Selective delayed response deficits in Parkinson's and Alzheimer's disease. *Archives of Neurology, 43,* 886–890.

Gerstmann, J. (1940). Syndrome of finger agnosia, disorientation for right and left, agraphia and acalculia. *Archives of Neurology and Psychiatry, 44,* 398–408.

Geschwind, N. (1965). Disconnection syndromes in animals and man. *Brain, 88,* 237–294.

Geschwind, N. (1975). The apraxias: Neural mechanisms of disorders of learned movement. *American Scientist, 63,* 188–195.

Geschwind, N., & Kaplan, E. (1962). A human cerebral disconnection syndrome. *Neurology, 12,* 675–685.

Goldstein, K. H. (1944). The mental changes due to frontal lobe damage. *Journal of Psychology, 17,* 187–208.

Goodglass, H., & Kaplan, E. (1979). Assessment of cognitive deficit in the brain-injured patient. In M. S. Gazzaniga (Ed.), *Handbook of behavioral neurobiology:* Vol. 2. *Neuropsychology* (pp. 3–22). New York: Plenum Press.

Goodglass, H., & Kaplan, E. (1983). *The assessment of aphasia and related disorders.* Philadelphia: Lea & Febiger.

Head, H. (1926). Aphasia and kindred disorders of speech. New York: Macmillan.

Heaton, R. K. (1981). *Wisconsin Card Sorting Test Manual.* Odessa, Fla.: Psychological Assessment Resources.

Heilman, K. M., Watson, R. T., & Valenstein, E. (1985). Neglect and related disorders. In K. M. Heilman & E. Valenstein (Eds.), *Clinical Neuropsychology.* New York: Oxford University Press.

Heilman, K. M., & Valenstein, E. (1985). *Clinical neuropsychology* (2nd ed.). New York: Oxford University Press.

Henderson, V. W., Mack, W., & Williams, B. W. (1989). Spatial orientation in Alzheimer's disease. *Archives of Neurology, 46,* 391–394.

Huntzinger, J. A., Roosae, R. B., Schwartz, B. L., et al. (1992). Clock drawing in the screening-assessment of cognitive impairment in an ambulatory care setting: A preliminary report. *General Hospital Psychiatry, 14,* 142–144.

Jackson, J. H. (1874). On the nature of the duality of the brain. *Medical Press and Circular, 17, 19* (reprinted in *Brain,* 1915, *38,* 80–103).

Kaplan, E. (1988). A process approach to neuropsychological assessment. In T. Bull & B. K. Bryant (Eds.), *Clinical neuropsychology and brain function: Research, measurement, and practice* (pp. 129–167). Washington, D.C.: American Psychological Association.

Kaplan, E. (1990). The process approach to neurological assessment of psychiatric patients. *Journal of Neuropsychiatry, 2,* 72–87.

Kaplan, E., Fein, D., Morris, R., & Delis, D. C. (1991). *WAIS-R as a neuropsychological instrument. Manual.* San Antonio, Texas: The Psychological Corporation.

Kirk, A., & Kertesz, A. (1991). On drawing impairment in Alzheimer's disease. *Archives of Neurology, 48,* 73–77.

Kleist, K. (1912). Der gang und der gegenwartige stand der apraxieforschung. *Neurologie und Psychiatrie, 1,* 342–452.

Kolb, B., & Whishaw, I. (1990). *Fundamentals of human neuropsychology* (3rd ed.). New York: Freeman.

La Pointe, L. L., & Culton, G. L. (1969). Visual-spatial neglect subsequent to brain injury. *Journal of Speech and Hearing Disorders, 34,* 82–86.

Lees, A. J., & Smith, E. (1983). Cognitive deficits in early stages of Parkinson's disease. *Brain, 106,* 257–270.

Levin, H. S., Benton, A. L., & Grossman, R. G. (1982). *Neuropsychological consequences of closed head injury.* New York: Oxford University Press.

Lezak, M. (1983). *Neuropsychological assessment* (2nd ed.). New York: Oxford University Press.

Libon, D. J., Swenson, R., Barnoski, E., & Sands, L. T. (1993). Clock drawing as an assessment tool in dementia. *Archives of Clinical Neuropsychology, 8,* 405–416.

Luria, A. (1980). *Higher cortical functions in man* (2nd ed.). New York: Basic Books.

Mattis, S. (1988). *Dementia rating scale: Professional manual.* Odessa, Fla.: Psychological Assessment Resources.

Mayer-Gross, W. (1935). Some observations on apraxia. *Proceedings of the Royal Society of Medicine, 28,* 1203–1212.

McFie, J., & Zangwill, O. L. (1960). Visuo-constructive disabilities associated with lesions of the left cerebral hemisphere. *Brain, 83,* 243–260.

McKhann, G., Drachman, D., Folstein, M., Katzman, R., Price, D., & Stadlan, E. M. (1984). Clinical diagnosis of Alzheimer's disease: Report of NINCDS-ADRDA Work Group under auspices of Department of Health and Human Services Task Force on Alzheimer's disease. *Neurology, 34,* 939–944.

Mendez, M. F., Ala, T., & Underwood, K. L. (1992). Development of scoring criteria for the clock drawing task in Alzheimer's disease. *Journal of the American Geriatrics Society, 40,* 1095–1099.

Milner, B. (1958). Psychological defects produced by temporal lobe excision. *Research Publications of the Association for Research in Nervous and Mental Disease, 38,* 244–257.

Milner, B. (1966). Amnesia following operation on the temporal lobes. In C.W.M. Whitty & O. L. Zangwill (Eds.), *Amnesia* (pp. 109–133). London: Butterworths.

Montgomery, K., & Costa, L. (1983, February). *Neuropsychological test performance of a normal elderly sample.* Paper presented to the 11th annual meeting of the International Neuropsychological Society, Mexico City.

Moscovitch, M. (1989). Confabulation and the frontal system: Strategic vs associative retrieval in neuropsychological theories of memory. In H. L. Roediger III & F.I.M. Craik (Eds.), *Varieties of memory and consciousness: Essays in honor of Endel Tulving.* Hillsdale, N.J.: Erlbaum.

Moscovitch, M., & Winocur, G. (1992). Frontal lobes and memory. In L. R. Squire & D. L. Schacter (Eds.), *The encyclopedia of learning and memory* (pp. 182–186). New York: Macmillan.

Newcombe, F., Ratcliff, G., & Damasio, H. (1987). Dissociable impairments of visual and spatial processing following right posterior cerebral lesions: Clinical, neuropsychological, and anatomic evidence. *Neuropsychologia, 25,* 149–161.

Nussbaum, P. D., Fields, R. B., & Starratt, C. (1992). *Comparison of three scoring procedures for clock drawing.* Paper presented at the International Neuropsychological Society, San Diego.

Pattie, A. H., & Gilleard, C. J. (1975). A brief psychogeriatric assessment schedule: Validation against psychiatric diagnosis and discharge from hospital. *British Journal of Psychiatry, 127,* 489–493.

Piercy, M. F., & Smyth, V. (1962). Right hemisphere dominance for certain nonverbal intellectual skills. *Brain, 85,* 775–790.

Pincus, J. H., & Tucker, G. J. (1974). *Behavioral neurology.* New York: Oxford University Press.

Poppelreuter, W. (1917). *Die psychischen schadigungen durch kopfschuss im kriege 1914–1916 die storungen der niederen und hoheren schleistungen durch verletzungen des okzipitalhirns.* Leipzig: Voss.

Raven, J. D. (1965). *Guide to using the coloured progressive matrices.* London: H. K. Lewis.

Reason, J. T. (1979). Action not as planned. In G. Underwood & R. Stevens (Eds.), *Aspects of consciousness* (pp. 67–89). London: Academic Press.

Reisberg, B., Ferris, S. H., De Leon, M. J., et al. (1982). The global deterioration scale for assessment of primary degenerative dementia. *American Journal of Psychiatry, 139,* 1136–1139.

Rey, A. L. (1941). L'examen psychologique dans les cas d'encephalopathie traumatique. *Archives de Psychologie, 28,* 286–340.

Rouleau, I., Salmon, D. P., Butters, N., Kennedy, C., & McGuire, K. (1992). Quantitative and qualitative analyses of clock drawings in Alzheimer's and Huntington's disease. *Brain and Cognition, 18,* 70–87.

Schuell, H. (1965). *Differential diagnosis of aphasia with the Minnesota test.* Minneapolis: University of Minnesota Press.

Semmes, J., Weinstein, S., Ghent, L., & Teuber, H.-L. (1963). *Brain, 86,* 747–772.

Shallice, T. (1982). Specific impairment of planning. In D. E. Broadbent & L. Weiskrantz (Eds.), *The neuropsychology of cognitive function* (pp. 199–209). London: The Royal Society.

Shulman, K. I., Gold, D., Cohen, C., & Zucchero, C. (1993). Clock drawing and dementia in the community: A longitudinal study. *International Journal of Geriatric Psychiatry, 8,* 487–496.

Shulman, K., Sheldetsky, R., & Silver, I. (1986). The challenge of time: Clock-drawing and cognitive function in the elderly. *International Journal of Geriatric Psychiatry, 1,* 135–140.

Spreen, O., & Strauss, E. (1991). *A compendium of neuropsychological tests*. New York: Oxford University Press.

Strub, R. L., & Black, F. W. (1985). *The mental status examination in neurology* (2nd ed.). Philadelphia: F. A. Davis.

Stuss, D. T., & Benson, D. F. (1986). *The frontal lobes*. New York: Raven Press.

Sunderland, T., Hill, J. L., Mellow, A. M., Lawlor, B. A., Gundersheimer, J., Newhouse, P. A., & Grafman, J. F. (1989). *Journal of the American Geriatrics Society, 37,* 725–729.

Taylor, A. E., Saint-Cyr, J. A., & Lang, A. E. (1986). Frontal lobe dysfunction in Parkinson's disease. *Brain, 109,* 845–883.

Tuokko, H., Hadjistavropoulos, T., Miller, J. A., & Beattie, B. L. (1992). *Journal of the American Geriatrics Society, 40,* 579–584.

Van der Horst, L. (1934). Constructive apraxia: Psychological views on the conception of space. *Journal of Nervous and Mental Disease, 80,* 645–650.

Victor, M. (1979). Neurologic disorders due to alcoholism and malnutrition. In A. B. Baker & L. H. Baker (Eds.), *Clinical neurology* (Vol. 4). New York: Harper & Row.

Walsh, K. W. (1987). *Neuropsychology: A clinical approach* (2nd ed.). Edinburgh: Churchill Livingstone.

Warrington, E. K., James, M., & Kinsborne, M. (1966). Drawing disability in relation to laterality of cerebral lesion. *Brain, 89,* 53–82.

Warrington, E., & Rabin, P. (1970). Perceptual matching in patients with cerebral lesions. *Neuropsychologia, 8,* 53–82.

Wechsler, D. (1945). A standardized memory scale for clinical use. *Journal of Psychology, 19,* 87–95.

Wechsler, D. (1981). *Wechsler Adult Intelligence Scale—Revised*. San Antonio, Texas: The Psychological Corporation.

Weiner, W. J., & Lang, A. E. (1989). *Movement disorders: A comprehensive survey* (pp. 49–50). Mount Kisco, N.Y.: Futura Publishing Co.

Weintraub, S., & Mesulam, M.-M. (1985). Mental state assessment of young and and elderly adults in behavioral neurology. In M.-M. Mesulam (Ed.), *Principles of Behavioral Neurology*. Philadelphia: F. A. Davis.

Werner, H. (1937). Process and achievement: A basic problem of education and developmental psychology. *Harvard Educational Review, 7,* 353–368.

Werner, H. (1956). Microgenesis and aphasia. *Journal of Abnormal and Social Psychology, 52,* 343–353.

Williams, T. F. (1992, December). Report on panel crafting guidelines to help screen for dementia. *APA Monitor*, p. 4.

Winocur, G., & Moscovitch, M. (1990). A comparison of cognitive function in community-dwelling and institutionalized old people of normal intelligence. *Canadian Journal of Psychology, 44,* 435–444.

Wolf-Klein, G. P., Silverstone, F. A., Levy, A. P., & Brod, M. S. (1989). Screening for Alzheimer's disease by clock drawing. *Journal of the American Geriatrics Society, 37,* 730–736.

Appendix 1

Clock Drawing Questionnaire

1. Please indicate your primary specialty

	Please check
Geriatric Medicine	_____
Neurology	_____
Occupational Therapy	_____
Psychiatry	_____
Psychology	_____
Rehabilitation Medicine	_____
Speech Pathology	_____
Other (specify) _____	_____

2. Do you use a clock-drawing task in your clinical/research practice?

    a) clinical   yes ____   no ____

    b) research   yes ____   no ____

If answer to 1a and b is no, please indicate so and return in the enclosed self-addressed envelop.

If answer to 1a or b is yes, please answer the following questions.

3. For approximately how many years have you been using clock drawing in your

    a) clinical assessment?   _____

    b) research?   _____

4. How did you first learn of clock drawing as a cognitive measure?

    a) From a specific individual   yes ____   no ____

        If yes, who was it? _____

        _____

b) From the literature   yes ____   no ____

   If yes, please state source _____
   _____

c) Other (specify) _____   yes ____   no ____
   _____

5. How useful do you find clock drawing to contribute to

	not useful				very useful	N/A
	1	2	3	4	5	6
a) screening for cognitive impairment						
b) lesion localization						
c) diagnosis						
d) monitoring progression/ course of deficits/ disease						
e) research						
f) other (specify) _____						

6. When asking for a clock to be drawn, do you

a) Ask the patient to freely draw a   yes ____   no ____
   clock on a blank sheet of paper?

b) Ask the patient to put numbers on   yes ____   no ____   N/A ____
   the freely drawn clock?

c) Specify a time setting?   yes ____   no ____
   If yes, what time(s) is/are specified?
   _____

e) Ask the patient to copy a clock?   yes ____   no ____
   If yes, what time is the clock set
   to? _____

7. Comments:

Appendix 2

Comprehensive Scoring System

6:45 FREE-DRAWN CLOCK
Percentage of the Total Number of Subjects Who Made a Given Response

Circle

		Age Group						
		20-29	30-39	40-49	50-59	60-69	70-79	80-90
1. Clock contour drawn								
1) initially acceptable	1	100.0	95.0	97.4	100.0	96.0	96.3	87.8
2) acceptable after self-modification	2		5.0	2.6		4.0	3.7	12.2
3) no, unacceptable	3							
4) no, unacceptable even after attempt at self-modification	4							
5) no attempt made	5							
	n	40	40	39	52	75	54	41
If response to item 1 is 1) or 2) then complete items 2 and 3, otherwise skip to item 4.								
2. Clock contour is								
1) circular symmetrical	1	25.0	17.5	25.6	25.0	18.7	20.4	22.0
2) circular asymmetrical	2	57.5	47.5	48.7	57.7	64.0	57.4	51.2
3) horizontal oval-like symmetrical	3		5.0	7.7	3.8	1.3	1.9	
4) horizontal oval-like asymmetrical	4	2.5	7.5	7.7	5.8	4.0	7.4	22.0
5) vertical oval-like symmetrical	5	12.5	2.5		5.8	4.0	3.7	
6) vertical oval-like asymmetrical	6	2.5	17.5	10.3	1.9	5.3	7.4	4.9
7) other	7		2.5			2.7	1.9	
	n	40	40	39	52	75	54	41
3. Clock contour is								
1) too small to contain numbers	1							
2) overdrawn	2							
3) reproduced repeatedly	3							
4) closed	4	70.0	60.0	79.5	69.2	76.0	75.9	78.0
5) open	5	30.0	40.0	20.5	30.8	24.0	24.1	14.6
	1,4							4.9
	1,5							2.4
	n	40	40	39	52	75	54	41

Numbers

	20-29	30-39	40-49	50-59	60-69	70-79	80-90
4. Only numbers 1-12 all present							
1) yes	87.5	87.5	84.6	88.5	90.7	85.2	82.9
2) yes, after self-modification	10.0	10.0	15.4	7.7	6.7	7.4	12.2
3) no	2.5	2.5		1.9	1.3	1.9	4.9
4) no even after attempt at self-modification				1.9	1.3	5.6	
n	40	40	39	52	75	54	41

If response to item 4 is 1) or 2) then omit items 5 and 6.

	20-29	30-39	40-49	50-59	60-69	70-79	80-90
5. Able to make a reasonable attempt at numbers							
1) yes	100.0	100.0		100.0	100.0	100.0	100.0
2) no							
n	1	1		2	2	4	2
6. If more or less than all 12 numbers present							
1) numbers omitted due to space constraints (eg. circle too small)		100.0					
2) numbers omitted				50.0		50.0	50.0
3) numbers added						25.0	
4) numbers put in more than once consecutively (ie. perseverative)							
2,3,4	100.0			50.0	50.0	25.0	50.0
n	1	1		2	2	4	2
7. Number(s) representation							
1) as roman							2.4
2) as arabic	95.0	97.5	97.4	98.1	97.3	100.0	87.8
3) as words							
4) as strokes							
5) other							
2,4	5.0	2.5	2.6	1.9	2.7		9.8
n	40	40	39	52	75	54	41
8. Starting number(s)							
1) anchor numbers - 3,6,9,12 (any 2)	45.0	47.5	64.1	50.0	38.7	27.8	46.3
2) 12	50.0	45.0	20.5	40.4	54.7	61.1	41.5
3) 1	5.0	7.5	15.4	9.6	6.7	9.3	12.2
4) other						1.9	
n	40	40	39	52	75	54	41

	20-29	30-39	40-49	50-59	60-69	70-79	80-90
9. Direction of numbers written							
1) clockwise – numbers in correct order 1	95.0	100.0	100.0	98.1	100.0	96.3	97.6
2) clockwise – numbers in reverse order 2							
3) counterclockwise – numbers in correct order 3						1.9	
4) counterclockwise – numbers in reverse order 4							
1,3	2.5						
3,1	2.5			1.9		1.9	2.4
n	40	40	39	52	75	54	41
10. Rotated paper while drawing numbers							
1) yes 1						9.3	9.8
2) no 2	100.0	100.0	100.0	100.0	100.0	90.7	90.2
n	40	40	39	52	75	54	41
11. Number(s) oriented correctly							
1) yes 1	45.0	42.5	35.9	50.0	36.0	35.2	43.9
2) no 2	55.0	57.5	64.1	50.0	64.0	55.6	46.3
3) no, due to rotation of the paper while drawing number(s) 3						9.3	9.8
n	40	40	39	52	75	54	41
12. Numbers in the correct position							
1) Yes 1	97.5	100.0	97.4	96.2	82.7	72.2	75.6
2) No 2	2.5		2.6	3.8	17.3	27.8	24.4
n	40	40	39	52	75	54	41
13. Number(s) are written							
1) all numbers written horizontally across clock face							
2) some number(s) written horizontally across clock face							
3) all numbers written vertically across clock face							
4) some numbers written vertically across clock face							
5) 3 or more consecutive numbers written on a slope (not conforming to a circular configuration)							

	20-29	30-39	40-49	50-59	60-69	70-79	80-90
14. Numbers are at the periphery							
1) Yes	47.5	30.0	43.6	57.7	34.7	31.5	39.0
2) No	52.5	70.0	56.4	42.3	65.3	68.5	61.0
n	40	40	39	52	75	54	41
15. Numbers are situated							
1) all inside the clock	90.0	97.5	94.9	90.4	94.7	92.6	90.2
2) start on the inside and extend to the outside	2.5	2.5	5.1	5.8	1.3		2.4
3) all outside the clock	7.5			3.8	4.0	7.4	7.3
4) not applicable							
n	40	40	39	52	75	54	41
16. Numbers from 12-6/6-12 are evenly spaced							
1) yes/yes	7.5	20.0	7.7	13.5	14.7	7.4	12.2
2) yes/no	15.0	5.0	7.7	11.5	13.3	11.1	17.1
3) no/yes	10.0	10.0	33.3	23.1	18.7	16.7	12.2
4) no/no	67.5	65.0	51.3	51.9	53.3	64.8	58.5
n	40	40	39	52	75	54	41
17. Self-modifications							
1) orientation errors			2.6	1.9			2.4
2) starting number(s)						1.9	
3) direction of numbers		2.5					
4) sequence of numbers	2.5		2.6			1.9	
5) omission of numbers							
6) additional numbers							
7) numbers away from the periphery							4.9
8) spacing		5.0	5.1	3.8	5.3	7.4	4.9
9) no self-modifications	90.0	90.0	84.6	90.4	92.0	85.2	80.5
10) attempt at self modification yields incorrect numbers			2.6	1.9	1.3	1.9	2.4
11) self-modification of graphic representation of number(s)		2.5	2.6	1.9	1.3	1.9	
1,8	2.5						2.4
2,5	2.5						2.4
5,6	2.5						
2,8							
1,7							
8,11							
n	40	40	39	52	75	54	41

Hands

Definition of a hand: A line, with or without an arrow, directed toward a number.

18. Two hands present

	20-29	30-39	40-49	50-59	60-69	70-79	80-90
1) yes, initially	75.0	75.0	74.4	80.8	74.7	70.4	61.0
2) yes, after self-modification	22.5	22.5	25.6	13.5	16.0	14.8	19.5
3) no, 2 hands are not present						7.4	9.8
4) no, 2 hands are not present even after self-modification						1.9	
5) 2 hands are present but the time is incorrect	2.5	2.5		5.8	9.3	5.6	9.8
6) yes, but they are emanating from the 12 position of the clock							
n	40	40	39	52	75	54	41

If response to item 18 is 1), 2) or 6) then omit items 19 and 20.

19. Hour target number indicated by

	20-29	30-39	40-49	50-59	60-69	70-79	80-90
1) minute number written next to hour number (eg. a 10 written adjacent to the 11)						12.5	
2) a hand				33.3	42.9	50.0	37.5
3) otherwise marked						25.0	25.0
4) joined to the minute target number by one line						12.5	
5) hour target number not indicated	100.0	100.0		66.7	57.1		37.5
n	1	1		3	7	8	8

20. Minute target number indicated by

	20-29	30-39	40-49	50-59	60-69	70-79	80-90
1) a hand				66.7	28.6	12.5	
2) otherwise marked						12.5	12.5
3) joined to the hour target number by one line							
4) minute target number not indicated	100.0	100.0		33.3	71.4	75.0	87.5
n	1	1		3	7	8	8

21. Proportion of hands

	20-29	30-39	40-49	50-59	60-69	70-79	80-90
1) hour hand longer	5.0	10.0	10.3	19.2	18.7	22.2	19.5
2) minute hand longer	95.0	87.5	89.7	78.8	77.3	66.7	65.9
3) both hands the same length		2.5		1.9	2.7	1.9	
4) only one hand present						3.7	2.4
5) not applicable					1.3	5.6	12.2
n	40	40	39	52	75	54	41

For items 22 and 23 assign a negative value if the hand is displaced counterclockwise from the target number or a positive value if the hand is displaced clockwise from the target number. Not measured for Free and Pre-drawn clocks.

22. Displacement of hour hand/mark from target number in degrees

23. Displacement of minute hand/mark from target number in degrees

Items 24 and 25 are to be completed only if one or both of the target numbers are spatially incorrect.

24. Target number(s) are spatially incorrect but hour hand
   1) correctly pointing to the appropriate target number
   2) pointing to correct site
   3) not applicable - no hand(s) present
   4) pointing to the incorrect number and incorrect site

	20-29	30-39	40-49	50-59	60-69	70-79	80-90
1					40.0	40.0	28.6
2						20.0	14.3
3						20.0	14.3
4					20.0		28.6
1,2					40.0	20.0	14.3
n					5	5	7

25. Target number(s) are spatially incorrect but minute hand
   1) correctly pointing to the appropriate target number
   2) pointing to correct site
   3) not applicable - no hand(s) present
   4) pointing to the incorrect number and incorrect site

	20-29	30-39	40-49	50-59	60-69	70-79	80-90
1					40.0		28.6
2					20.0	20.0	14.3
3							14.3
4					20.0	80.0	28.6
1,2					20.0		14.3
n					5	5	7

26. Arrows on hands
   1) arrow on hour hand
   2) arrow on minute hand
   3) arrows on both hands
   4) arrows on neither hand
   5) not applicable - no hands

	20-29	30-39	40-49	50-59	60-69	70-79	80-90
1			2.6	1.9	1.3	5.6	7.3
2			2.6				
3	77.5	72.5	74.4	80.8	70.7	48.1	46.3
4	22.5	27.5	20.5	17.3	28.0	40.7	39.0
5						5.6	7.3
n	40	40	39	52	75	54	41

If response to item 26 is 4) or 5) then omit items 27 and 28.
N.B.(3 mm = 1/8 inch, 6 mm = 1/4 inch)

	20-29	30-39	40-49	50-59	60-69	70-79	80-90
27. Arrows are displaced from hands by							
1) no displacement	54.8	86.2	58.1	72.1	64.8	82.8	86.4
2) ≤ 4 mm	45.2	13.8	41.9	27.9	35.2	17.2	13.6
3) > 4 mm and ≤ 6 mm							
4) > 6 mm							
n	31	29	31	43	54	29	22
28. Arrows on hands pointing in the wrong direction							
1) yes					1.9	6.9	
2) no	100.0	100.0	100.0	100.0	98.1	93.1	100.0
n	31	29	31	43	54	29	22
29. Any superfluous markings on the clock							
1) yes	2.5	2.5	2.6	3.8	9.3	13.0	12.2
2) no	97.5	97.5	97.4	96.2	90.7	87.0	87.8
n	40	40	39	52	75	54	41
If response to item 29 is 2) then omit items 30 and 31.							
30. Superfluous lines							
1) emanating from 12 position of clock						25.0	33.3
2) 3 hands present							33.3
3) other superfluous lines							
4) spokes of a wheel drawn on part of the clock					100.0	25.0	
5) spokes of a wheel drawn on the whole clock						25.0	
1,2							
1,3						25.0	33.3
n					1	4	3
31. Miscellaneous markings							
1) time is written across clock face							
2) time is written outside of the circle							
3) picture of a human face is drawn on clock							
4) hands with fingers							
5) markings such as words							
6) other	100.0	100.0	100.0	100.0	100.0	100.0	100.0
n	1	1	1	2	7	4	3

	20-29	30-39	40-49	50-59	60-69	70-79	80-90
Joining of Hands							
32. Both hands joined							
1) yes	65.0	75.0	61.5	61.5	54.7	63.3	70.3
2) no, mild (<3 mm apart)	30.0	22.5	30.8	28.8	33.3	28.6	21.6
3) no, moderate (3 mm – 12 mm apart)	2.5	2.5	5.1	3.8	4.0	4.1	8.1
4) no, severe (>12 mm apart)						4.1	
5) yes, but not at the ends	2.5		2.6	5.8	8.0		
n	40	40	39	52	75	49	37

N.B. (3 mm = 1/8 inch, 12 mm = 1/2 inch)

If response to item 32 is 1) or 5) then omit item 33.

	20-29	30-39	40-49	50-59	60-69	70-79	80-90
33. Hands are not joined							
1) hour hand only emanates from subject's drawn center	38.5	40.0	14.3	17.6	14.3	11.1	27.3
2) minute hand only emanates from subject's drawn center	23.1	20.0	35.7	23.5	25.0	27.8	18.2
3) neither hand emanates from subject's drawn center	23.1	20.0	28.6	41.2	28.6	27.8	36.4
4) not applicable (subject did not draw a center)	15.4	20.0	21.4	17.6	32.1	33.3	18.2
n	13	10	14	17	28	18	11

<u>Center</u> – If hands are not joined then extrapolate them to create a center for purposes of measurement.

	20-29	30-39	40-49	50-59	60-69	70-79	80-90
34. Center is drawn by subject							
1) yes	82.5	80.0	69.2	73.1	65.3	61.1	68.3
2) no, but a center can be extrapolated/ inferred by the point at which the hands are joined or by extrapolating the ends of two hands which are not joined	17.5	20.0	30.8	26.9	34.7	31.5	24.4
3) no, the hands are not joined, and the distance between the ends of the hands is too great to extrapolate a center or there are not two hands						7.5	7.3
n	40	40	39	52	75	54	41

If response to item 34 is 2) or 3) then omit items 35–38. Items 35, 36, and 38 not calculated for Free and Pre-drawn clocks.

35. Distance of subject's center from
    vertical axis (in millimeters).
    The measurement is assigned a positive
    value if right of the axis or a negative
    value if left of the axis.

36. Distance of subject's center from
    horizontal axis (in millimeters).
    The measurement is assigned a positive
    value if above the axis or a negative value
    if below the axis.

37. Subject's drawn center is in

		20-29	30-39	40-49	50-59	60-69	70-79	80-90
1)	upper right	15.2	28.1	25.9	15.8	16.3	12.1	17.9
2)	upper left	18.2	18.8	22.2	15.8	26.5	9.1	7.1
3)	lower right	12.1	21.9	14.8	5.3	6.1	6.1	14.3
4)	lower left	24.2	12.5	7.4	13.2	8.2	12.1	7.1
5)	right axis	3.0		3.7	5.3	10.2	9.1	7.1
6)	left axis			7.4	13.2	6.1	18.2	25.0
7)	top axis	21.2	9.4	14.8	13.2		9.1	3.6
8)	bottom axis	3.0	6.2		2.6	10.2	3.0	3.6
9)	center	3.0	3.1	3.7	15.8	16.3	21.2	14.3
n		33	32	27	38	49	33	28

38. Distance from examiner's center to subject's center
    (in millimeters).

If response to item 34 is 2) then complete
items 39-43.

39. A center can be either inferred by the
    point at which the hands are joined or
    by extrapolating the ends of two hands
    which are not joined

		20-29	30-39	40-49	50-59	60-69	70-79	80-90
1)	yes, a center can be inferred from the point of joining of the hands	77.8	70.0	64.3	75.0	67.9	68.7	71.4
2)	yes, a center can be extrapolated from the ends of two hands that are not joined	22.2	30.0	35.7	25.0	32.1	31.3	28.6
n		9	10	14	16	28	16	14

	20-29	30-39	40-49	50-59	60-69	70-79	80-90
1	11.1	40.0	21.4	18.8	10.7	18.8	14.3
2	55.6	10.0	21.4	31.3	10.7	12.5	35.7
3	11.1		28.6		17.9	6.2	14.3
4	22.2	20.0	7.1	25.0	28.6	31.3	21.4
5		10.0	14.3	12.5	7.1	6.2	14.3
6		20.0		6.2	17.9	18.8	
7							
8			7.1	6.2	3.6	6.2	
9					3.6		
n	9	10	14	16	28	16	14

40. Distance of inferred/extrapolated center from vertical axis (in millimeters). The measurement is assigned a positive value if right of the axis or a negative value if left of the axis. Not calculated for Free and Pre-drawn clocks.

41. Distance of inferred/extrapolated center from the horizontal axis (in millimeters). The measurement is assigned a positive value if above the axis or a negative value if below the axis. Not calculated for Free and Pre-drawn clocks.

42. Inferred/extrapolated center is in
1) upper right
2) upper left
3) lower right
4) lower left
5) right axis
6) left axis
7) top axis
8) bottom axis
9) center

43. Distance from examiner's center to inferred/extrapolated center (in millimeters). Not calculated for Free and Pre-drawn clocks.

6:05 PRE-DRAWN CLOCK

Percentage of the Total Number of
Subjects Who Made a Given Response

Items 1-3 do not apply to pre-drawn clock

Numbers

		Age Group						
		20-29	30-39	40-49	50-59	60-69	70-79	80-90
4. Only numbers 1-12 all present								
1) yes	1	97.5	90.0	87.2	88.5	90.8	84.7	70.7
2) yes, after self-modification	2	2.5	10.0	5.1	5.8	3.9	6.8	19.5
3) no	3			7.7	5.8	3.9	6.8	9.8
4) no even after attempt at self-modification	4					1.3	1.7	
	n	40	40	39	52	76	59	41

If response to item 4 is 1) or 2) then omit items 5 and 6.

		20-29	30-39	40-49	50-59	60-69	70-79	80-90
5. Able to make a reasonable attempt at numbers								
1) yes	1			100.0	100.0	100.0	100.0	100.0
2) no	2							
	n			3	3	4	5	4
6. If more or less than all 12 numbers present								
1) numbers omitted due to space constraints (eg. circle too small)	1							
2) numbers omitted	2				66.7	25.0	60.0	25.0
3) numbers added	3					25.0	20.0	25.0
4) numbers put in more than once consecutively (ie. perseverative)	4							
	2,3					25.0	20.0	25.0
	2,3,4			100.0	33.3	25.0		25.0
	n			3	3	4	5	4
7. Number(s) representation								
1) as roman	1							2.4
2) as arabic	2	92.5	100.0	97.4	96.2	97.4	100.0	87.8
3) as words	3							
4) as strokes	4							
5) other	5	7.5		2.6	1.9	2.6		9.8
	2,4							
	2,5				1.9			
	n	40	40	39	52	76	59	41

		20-29	30-39	40-49	50-59	60-69	70-79	80-90
8.	**Starting number(s)**							
	1) anchor numbers – 3,6,9,12 (any two)	52.5	52.5	74.4	63.5	52.6	45.8	58.5
	2) 12	47.5	42.5	20.5	28.8	43.4	47.5	39.0
	3) 1		5.0	5.1	7.7	3.9	6.8	2.4
	4) other							
	n	40	40	39	52	76	59	41
9.	**Direction of numbers written**							
	1) clockwise – numbers in correct order	95.0	95.0	100.0	96.2	96.1	94.9	92.7
	2) clockwise – numbers in reverse order							2.4
	3) counterclockwise – numbers in correct order	2.5				1.3		2.4
	4) counterclockwise – numbers in reverse order							
	3,1	2.5	5.0		1.9	2.6	1.7	2.4
	1,3				1.9		3.4	
	n	40	40	39	52	76	59	41
10.	**Rotated paper while drawing numbers**							
	1) yes						6.8	12.2
	2) no	100.0	100.0	100.0	100.0	100.0	93.2	87.8
	n	40	40	39	52	76	59	41
11.	**Number(s) oriented correctly**							
	1) yes	40.0	35.0	25.6	48.1	42.1	37.3	29.3
	2) no	60.0	65.0	74.4	51.9	57.9	55.9	58.5
	3) no, due to rotation of the paper while drawing number(s)						6.8	12.2
	n	40	40	39	52	76	59	41
12.	**Numbers in the correct position**							
	1) Yes	97.5	95.0	92.3	98.1	86.8	74.6	63.4
	2) No	2.5	5.0	7.7	1.9	13.2	25.4	36.6
	n	40	40	39	52	76	59	41

		20-29	30-39	40-49	50-59	60-69	70-79	80-90
13.	**Number(s) are written**							
	1) all numbers written horizontally across clock face							
	2) some number(s) written horizontally across clock face							
	3) all numbers written vertically across clock face							
	4) some numbers written vertically across clock face							
	5) 3 or more consecutive numbers written on a slope (not conforming to a circular configuration)							
14.	**Numbers are at the periphery**							
	1) Yes	30.0	27.5	38.5	51.9	47.4	39.0	36.6
	2) No	70.0	72.5	61.5	48.1	52.6	61.0	63.4
	n	40	40	39	52	76	59	41
15.	**Numbers are situated**							
	1) all inside the clock	90.0	97.5	92.3	92.3	93.4	93.2	87.8
	2) start on the inside and extend to the outside	2.5		2.6	3.8	1.3		2.4
	3) all outside the clock	7.5	2.5	5.1	3.8	5.3	6.8	9.8
	4) not applicable							
	n	40	40	39	52	76	59	41
16.	**Numbers from 12-6/6-12 are evenly spaced**							
	1) yes/yes	12.5	22.5	15.4	19.2	21.1	8.5	14.6
	2) yes/no	22.5	7.5	17.9	11.5	15.8	16.9	7.3
	3) no/yes	15.0	27.5	28.2	25.0	19.7	23.7	12.2
	4) no/no	50.0	42.5	38.5	44.2	43.4	50.8	65.9
	n	40	40	39	52	76	59	41

17. Self-modifications

	20-29	30-39	40-49	50-59	60-69	70-79	80-90
1							7.3
2							
3							
4							
5							
6							
7							
8	2.5	5.0	2.6	3.8	5.3	10.2	17.1
9	97.5	90.0	94.9	92.3	92.1	84.7	75.6
10							
11		2.5	2.6	1.9	1.3	1.7	
2,8						1.7	
5,6						1.7	
2,5		2.5					
5,8				1.9			
7,8					1.3		
8,10							
n	40	40	39	52	76	59	41

17. Self-modifications
   1) orientation errors
   2) starting number(s)
   3) direction of numbers
   4) sequence of numbers
   5) omission of numbers
   6) additional numbers
   7) numbers away from the periphery
   8) spacing
   9) no self-modifications
   10) attempt at self modification yields incorrect numbers
   11) self-modification of graphic representation of number(s)

Hands

Definition of a hand: A line, with or without an arrow, directed toward a number.

18. Two hands present

	20-29	30-39	40-49	50-59	60-69	70-79	80-90
1	95.0	87.5	84.6	84.6	92.1	78.0	73.2
2	5.0	12.5	15.4	11.5	5.3	5.1	12.2
3						10.2	9.8
4							
5				3.8	1.3	6.8	4.9
6					1.3		
n	40	40	39	52	76	59	41

18. Two hands present
   1) yes, initially
   2) yes, after self-modification
   3) no, 2 hands are not present
   4) no, 2 hands are not present even after self-modification
   5) 2 hands are present but the time is incorrect
   6) yes, but they are emanating from the 12 position of the clock

If response in item 18 is 1), 2) or 6) then omit items 19 and 20.

19. Hour target number indicated by

	20-29	30-39	40-49	50-59	60-69	70-79	80-90
1) minute number written next to hour number (eg. a 10 written adjacent to the 11)							
2) a hand				100.0	100.0	40.0	50.0
3) otherwise marked						30.0	50.0
4) joined to the minute target number by one line						10.0	
5) hour target number not indicated						20.0	
n				2	1	10	6

20. Minute target number indicated by

	20-29	30-39	40-49	50-59	60-69	70-79	80-90
1) a hand							
2) otherwise marked						20.0	16.7
3) joined to the hour target number by one line						10.0	
4) minute target number not indicated				100.0	100.0	70.0	83.3
n				2	1	10	6

21. Proportion of hands

	20-29	30-39	40-49	50-59	60-69	70-79	80-90
1) hour hand longer	5.0	15.0	10.3	19.2	26.3	35.6	39.0
2) minute hand longer	92.5	85.0	89.7	80.8	73.7	50.8	51.2
3) both hands the same length	2.5					3.4	2.4
4) only one hand present						3.4	7.3
5) not applicable						6.8	
n	40	40	39	52	76	59	41

For items 22 and 23 assign a negative value if the hand is displaced counterclockwise from the target number or a positive value if the hand is displaced clockwise from the target number. Not measured for Free and Pre-drawn clocks.

22. Displacement of hour hand/mark from target number in degrees

23. Displacement of minute hand/mark from target number in degrees

Items 24 and 25 are to be completed for the Free Drawn Clock and Pre-drawn circle condition only if one or both of the target numbers are spatially incorrect.

	20-29	30-39	40-49	50-59	60-69	70-79	80-90
24. Target number(s) are spatially incorrect but hour hand							
1) correctly pointing to the appropriate target number						37.5	37.5
2) pointing to correct site						12.5	12.5
3) not applicable - no hand(s) present						12.5	12.5
4) pointing to the incorrect number and incorrect site						37.5	37.5
1,2					100.0		
n					1	8	8
25. Target number(s) are spatially incorrect but minute hand							
1) correctly pointing to the appropriate target number						37.5	25.0
2) pointing to correct site						12.5	12.5
3) not applicable - no hand(s) present						25.0	12.5
4) pointing to the incorrect number and incorrect site						12.5	50.0
1,2					100.0		
n					1	8	8
26. Arrows on hands							
1) arrow on hour hand					1.3	6.8	7.3
2) arrow on minute hand		2.5		1.9	5.3	3.4	2.4
3) arrows on both hands	77.5	67.5	76.9	78.8	69.7	49.2	53.7
4) arrows on neither hand	22.5	30.0	23.1	19.2	23.7	33.9	29.3
5) not applicable - no hands						6.8	7.3
n	40	40	39	52	76	59	41
27. Arrows are displaced from hands by							
1) no displacement	51.6	67.9	63.3	66.7	70.7	68.6	73.1
2) ≤ 4 mm	45.2	32.1	33.3	33.3	29.3	31.4	26.9
3) > 4 mm and ≤ 6 mm	3.2		3.3				
4) > 6 mm							
n	31	28	30	42	58	35	26

If response to item 26 is 4) or 5) then omit items 27 and 28.

N.B.(3 mm = 1/8 inch, 6 mm = 1/4 inch)

	20-29	30-39	40-49	50-59	60-69	70-79	80-90
28. Arrows on hands pointing in the wrong direction							
1) yes	100.0	100.0	100.0	100.0	1.7	5.7	100.0
2) no					98.3	94.3	
n	31	28	30	42	58	35	26
29. Any superfluous markings on the clock							
1) yes		2.5	7.7	3.8	2.6	10.2	7.3
2) no	100.0	97.5	92.3	96.2	97.4	89.8	92.7
n	40	40	39	52	76	59	41

If response to item 29 is 2) then omit items 30 and 31.

	20-29	30-39	40-49	50-59	60-69	70-79	80-90
30. Superfluous lines							
1) emanating from 12 position of clock		100.0		100.0	100.0	66.7	50.0
2) 3 hands present							
3) other superfluous lines							
4) spokes of a wheel drawn on part of the clock							
5) spokes of a wheel drawn on the whole clock						33.3	
1,2							50.0
1,3							
n		1		1	2	3	2
31. Miscellaneous markings							
1) time is written across clock face		100.0	33.3	100.0	100.0	100.0	50.0
2) time is written outside of the circle							
3) picture of a human face is drawn on clock							
4) hands with fingers							
5) markings such as words							
6) other			66.7				50.0
1,6							
n		1	3	1	2	3	2

Joining of Hands

	20-29	30-39	40-49	50-59	60-69	70-79	80-90
32. Both hands joined							
1) yes	60.0	40.0	46.2	32.7	38.2	35.8	40.5
2) no, mild (<3 mm apart)	32.5	40.0	41.0	42.3	38.2	45.3	45.9
3) no, moderate (3 mm - 12 mm apart)	7.5	15.0	12.8	23.1	19.7	13.2	13.5
4) no, severe (>12 mm apart)		5.0			2.6	5.7	
5) yes, but not at the ends				1.9	1.3		
n	40	40	39	52	76	53	37

N.B.(3 mm = 1/8 inch, 12 mm = 1/2 inch)

If response to item 32 is 1) or 5) then omit
item 33.

		20-29	30-39	40-49	50-59	60-69	70-79	80-90
33.	Hands are not joined							
	1) hour hand only emanates from subject's drawn center	1	25.0	12.5	33.3	11.8	15.2	27.3	22.7
	2) minute hand only emanates from subject's drawn center	2	18.8	37.5	19.0	38.2	30.4	18.2	22.7
	3) neither hand emanates from subject's drawn center	3	31.3	20.8	23.8	41.2	37.0	24.2	22.7
	4) not applicable (subject did not draw a center)	4	25.0	29.2	23.8	8.8	17.4	30.3	31.8
		n	16	24	21	34	46	33	22
Center – If hands are not joined then extrapolate them to create a center for purposes of measurement.									
34.	Center is drawn by subject								
	1) yes	1	72.5	72.5	69.2	84.6	73.7	64.4	70.7
	2) no, but a center can be extrapolated/ inferred by the point at which the hands are joined or by extrapolating the ends of two hands which are not joined	2	27.5	27.5	30.8	15.4	23.7	25.4	24.4
	3) no, the hands are not joined, and the distance between the ends of the hands is too great to extrapolate a center or there are not two hands	3					2.6	10.2	4.9
		n	40	40	39	52	76	59	41

If response to item 34 is 2) or 3) then
omit items 35-38. Items 35, 36 and 38 not
calculated for Free and Pre-drawn
clocks.

35. Distance of subject's center from
vertical axis (in millimeters).
The measurement is assigned a positive
value if right of the axis or a negative
value if left of the axis.

36. Distance of subject's center from
horizontal axis (in millimeters).
The measurement is assigned a positive
value if above the axis or a negative value
if below the axis.

	20-29	30-39	40-49	50-59	60-69	70-79	80-90
1	10.3	31.0	14.8	4.5	33.3	13.2	20.7
2	10.3	17.2	29.6	20.5	7.0	21.1	13.8
3	10.3	3.4	18.5	11.4	14.0	18.4	3.4
4	27.6	20.7	25.9	4.5	8.8	5.3	6.9
5	3.4	3.4			3.5	5.3	3.4
6		3.4	3.7	22.7		5.3	10.3
7	20.7	10.3		13.6	17.5	15.8	31.0
8	3.4	3.4		6.8	5.3	2.6	3.4
9	13.8	6.9	7.4	15.9	10.5	13.2	6.9
n	29	29	27	44	57	38	29

	20-29	30-39	40-49	50-59	60-69	70-79	80-90
1	63.6	38.5	58.3	45.5	47.4	37.5	27.3
2	36.4	61.5	41.7	54.5	52.6	62.5	72.7
n	11	13	12	11	19	16	11

37. Subject's drawn center is in
   1) upper right
   2) upper left
   3) lower right
   4) lower left
   5) right axis
   6) left axis
   7) top axis
   8) bottom axis
   9) center

38. Distance from examiner's center to subject's center (in millimeters).

If response to item 34 is 2) then complete items 39-43.

39. A center can be either inferred by the point at which the hands are joined or by extrapolating the ends of two hands which are not joined
   1) yes, a center can be inferred from the point of joining of the hands
   2) yes, a center can be extrapolated from the ends of two hands that are not joined

40. Distance of inferred/extrapolated center from vertical axis (in millimeters). The measurement is assigned a positive value if right of the axis or a negative value if left of the axis. Not calculated for Free and Pre-drawn clocks.

41. Distance of inferred/extrapolated center from the horizontal axis (in millimeters). The measurement is assigned a positive value if above the axis or a negative value if below the axis. Not calculated for Free and Pre-drawn clocks.

42. Inferred/extrapolated center is in

		20-29	30-39	40-49	50-59	60-69	70-79	80-90
1)	upper right	9.1	38.5	41.7	18.2	31.6	50.0	36.4
2)	upper left	18.2	30.8	25.0	27.3	5.3	12.5	27.3
3)	lower right	27.3			9.1	21.1		9.1
4)	lower left	18.2	23.1	16.7	9.1	15.8	25.0	
5)	right axis	9.1		8.3		10.5		
6)	left axis				9.1			
7)	top axis			8.3				
8)	bottom axis	18.2	7.7		9.1	5.3	12.5	9.1
9)	center				18.2	10.5		18.2
n		11	13	12	11	19	16	11

43. Distance from examiner's center to inferred/
    extrapolated center (in millimeters). Not
    calculated for Free and Pre-drawn clocks.

11:10-EXAMINER CLOCK
Percentage of the Total Number of Subjects Who Made a Given Response

Items 1-17 do not apply to examiner clocks

Hands

Definition of a hand: A line, with or without an arrow, directed toward a number.

18. Two hands present
    1) yes, initially
    2) yes, after self-modification
    3) no, 2 hands are not present
    4) no, 2 hands are not present even after self-modification
    5) 2 hands are present but the time is incorrect
    6) yes, but they are emanating from the 12 position of the clock

If response in item 18 is 1), 2) or 6) then omit items 19 and 20.

19. Hour target number indicated by
    1) minute number written next to hour number (eg. a 10 written adjacent to the 11)
    2) a hand
    3) otherwise marked
    4) joined to the minute target number by one line
    5) hour target number not indicated

20. Minute target number indicated by
    1) a hand
    2) otherwise marked
    3) joined to the hour target number by one line
    4) minute target number not indicated

				Age Group			
	20-29	30-39	40-49	50-59	60-69	70-79	80-90
18.							
1	97.5	92.5	90.0	78.8	88.2	78.0	70.7
2	2.5	5.0	10.0	17.3	9.2	6.8	17.1
3		2.5			1.3	6.8	12.2
4						1.7	
5				3.8	1.3	6.8	
6							
n	40	40	40	52	76	59	41
19.							
1						11.1	20.0
2				100.0		33.3	
3						33.3	
4					50.0	11.1	60.0
5		100.0			50.0	11.1	20.0
2,3							
1,3							
n		1		2	2	9	5
20.							
1					50.0	11.1	20.0
2						11.1	
3				100.0	50.0		
4		100.0				77.8	80.0
n		1		2	2	9	5

21. Proportion of hands

	20-29	30-39	40-49	50-59	60-69	70-79	80-90
1) hour hand longer	2.5	7.5		13.5	14.5	11.9	34.1
2) minute hand longer	97.5	90.0	100.0	86.5	82.9	74.6	53.7
3) both hands the same length		2.5			1.3	5.1	2.4
4) only one hand present					1.3	3.4	9.8
5) not applicable						5.1	
n	40	40	40	52	76	59	41

For items 22 and 23 assign a negative value if the hand is displaced counterclockwise from the target number or a positive value if the hand is displaced clockwise from the target number.

22. Displacement of hour hand/mark from target number in degrees

	20-29	30-39	40-49	50-59	60-69	70-79	80-90
≥-15							
-12		2.5					
-9	2.5	2.5	2.5		1.3		
-6	2.5	12.5	2.5	1.9	1.3	1.7	2.4
-3	2.5	12.5	20.0	1.9	6.6	5.1	4.9
0	52.5	40.0	25.0	36.5	47.4	52.5	26.8
+3	22.5	10.0	17.5	23.1	14.5	8.5	14.6
+6	10.0	12.5	20.0	21.2	21.1	16.9	24.4
+9	7.5	7.5	7.5	5.8	6.6	6.8	4.9
+12			5.0	7.7	1.3	6.8	22.0
+15				1.9		1.7	
n	40	40	40	52	76	59	41

23. Displacement of minute hand/mark from target number in degrees

	20-29	30-39	40-49	50-59	60-69	70-79	80-90
≥-30				3.8			
-15							
-12							
-9			2.5			7.2	
-6		7.5	15.0			1.8	2.4
-3	10.0	32.5	25.0	5.8	2.6	1.8	4.9
0	50.0	47.5	32.5	50.0	60.5	46.4	26.3
+3	35.0	12.5	20.0	15.4	17.1	17.9	14.6
+6	5.0		5.0	23.1	18.4	17.9	24.4
+9				1.9	1.3	3.6	4.9
+12						3.6	22.0
+15							
+30							
n	40	40	40	52	76	56	37

Items 24 and 25 are to be completed for the Free Drawn Clock and Pre-drawn circle condition only if one or both of the target numbers are spatially incorrect. Items 24 and 25 do not apply to Examiner clocks.

	20-29	30-39	40-49	50-59	60-69	70-79	80-90
26. Arrows on hands							
1) arrow on hour hand			2.5	1.9	2.6	3.4	9.8
2) arrow on minute hand					1.3		
3) arrows on both hands	77.5	65.0	75.0	76.9	72.4	50.8	43.9
4) arrows on neither hand	22.5	35.0	22.5	21.2	23.7	40.7	36.6
5) not applicable - no hands						5.1	9.8
n	40	40	40	52	76	59	41

If response to item 26 is 4) or 5) then omit items 27 and 28.
N.B.(3 mm = 1/8 inch, 6 mm = 1/4 inch)

	20-29	30-39	40-49	50-59	60-69	70-79	80-90
27. Arrows are displaced from hands by							
1) no displacement	41.9	69.2	51.6	53.7	63.8	75.0	81.8
2) ≤ 4 mm	54.8	30.8	45.2	46.3	36.2	21.9	18.2
3) > 4 mm and ≤ 6 mm	3.2		3.2			3.1	
4) > 6 mm							
n	31	26	31	41	58	32	22

	20-29	30-39	40-49	50-59	60-69	70-79	80-90
28. Arrows on hands pointing in the wrong direction							
1) yes						6.2	4.5
2) no	100.0	100.0	100.0	100.0	100.0	93.7	95.5
n	31	26	31	41	58	32	22

	20-29	30-39	40-49	50-59	60-69	70-79	80-90
29. Any superfluous markings on the clock							
1) yes		2.5	5.0		5.3	5.1	
2) no	100.0	97.5	95.0	100.0	94.7	94.9	100.0
n	40	40	40	52	76	59	41

If response to item 29 is 2) then omit items 30 and 31.

	20-29	30-39	40-49	50-59	60-69	70-79	80-90
30. Superfluous lines							
1) emanating from 12 position of clock		100.0				50.0	
2) 3 hands present							
3) other superfluous lines							
4) spokes of a wheel drawn on part of the clock					100.0	50.0	
5) spokes of a wheel drawn on the whole clock							
n		1			2	2	

	20-29	30-39	40-49	50-59	60-69	70-79	80-90
31. Miscellaneous markings							
1) time is written across clock face							
2) time is written outside of the circle							
3) picture of a human face is drawn on clock			50.0				
4) hands with fingers							
5) markings such as words							
6) other			50.0		100.0	100.0	
n			2		2	1	
Joining of Hands							
32. Both hands joined							
1) yes	65.0	59.0	52.5	61.5	38.7	44.4	47.2
2) no, mild (<3 mm apart)	27.5	25.6	35.0	23.1	40.0	29.6	25.0
3) no, moderate (3 mm - 12 mm apart)	2.5	7.7	5.0	5.8	14.7	16.7	19.4
4) no, severe (>12 mm apart)		2.6		1.9	1.3	5.6	
5) yes, but not at the ends	5.0	5.1	7.5	7.7	5.3	3.7	8.3
n	40	39	40	52	75	54	36

N.B. (3 mm = 1/8 inch, 12 mm = 1/2 inch)

If response to item 32 is 1) or 5) then omit item 33.

	20-29	30-39	40-49	50-59	60-69	70-79	80-90
33. Hands are not joined							
1) hour hand only emanates from subject's drawn center	41.7	28.6	31.3	12.5	38.1	25.0	12.5
2) minute hand only emanates from subject's drawn center	16.7	14.3	6.2	31.3	19.0	17.9	25.0
3) neither hand emanates from subject's drawn center	25.0	14.3	31.3	37.5	28.6	32.1	43.8
4) not applicable (subject did not draw a center)	16.7	42.9	31.3	18.8	14.3	25.0	18.8
n	12	14	16	16	42	28	16

Center - If hands are not joined then
extrapolate them to create a center
for purposes of measurement.

34. Center is drawn by subject

1) yes
2) no, but a center can be extrapolated/
   inferred by the point at which the
   hands are joined or by extrapolating
   the ends of two hands which are
   not joined
3) no, the hands are not joined, the
   distance between the ends of two hands
   is too great to extrapolate a center,
   or there are not two hands

If response to item 34 is 2) or 3) then
omit items 35-38.

35. Mean distance of subject's center from
    vertical axis (in millimeters).
    The measurement is assigned a positive
    value if right of the axis or a negative
    value if left of the axis.

36. Mean distance of subject's center from
    horizontal axis (in millimeters).
    The measurement is assigned a positive
    value if above the axis or a negative
    value if below the axis.

37. Subject's drawn center is in

1) upper right
2) upper left
3) lower right
4) lower left
5) right axis
6) left axis
7) top axis
8) bottom axis
9) center

		20-29	30-39	40-49	50-59	60-69	70-79	80-90
34	1	82.5	67.5	70.0	82.7	78.9	59.3	73.2
	2	17.5	27.5	30.0	17.3	18.4	27.1	17.1
	3		5.0			2.6	13.6	9.8
	n	40	40	40	52	76	59	41
35	X̄	-1.0	.4	-.5	-.3	.2	.4	-.3
	SD	1.7	1.5	1.6	1.7	2.2	2.2	3.1
	n	33	27	28	43	61	35	30
36	X̄	.2	1.4	.2	.9	.9	1.0	1.3
	SD	3.0	3.4	3.3	3.2	2.6	2.7	2.5
	n	33	27	28	43	61	35	30
37	1	12.1	33.3	10.7	9.3	26.2	28.6	16.7
	2	27.3	14.8	17.9	23.3	13.1	25.7	20.0
	3	6.1	3.7	3.6	11.6	11.5	11.4	6.7
	4	30.3	7.4	28.6	11.6	8.2	5.7	6.7
	5	3.0	18.5	7.1	4.7	16.4	5.7	13.3
	6	6.1	7.4	7.1	11.6	8.2	5.7	6.7
	7	6.1	3.7	7.1	11.6	8.2	5.7	13.3
	8	3.0	3.7	7.1	7.0	3.3		3.3
	9	6.1	7.4	3.6	9.3	4.9	11.4	13.3
	n	33	27	28	43	61	35	30

	20-29	30-39	40-49	50-59	60-69	70-79	80-90
X̄	3.1	2.5	2.9	2.7	2.8	2.9	2.8
SD	1.9	3.0	2.3	2.6	2.3	2.1	3.1
n	33	27	28	43	61	35	30
1	55.6	50.0	46.7	75.0	43.7	70.6	54.5
2	44.4	50.0	53.3	25.0	56.2	29.4	45.5
n	9	12	15	12	16	17	11
X̄	-1.3	.2	.1	.5	1.1	.4	1.0
SD	2.2	3.2	3.2	2.4	3.2	2.9	5.4
n	9	12	15	12	16	17	11
X̄	2.2	-1.5	1.6	-.9	4.0	1.3	3.4
SD	6.7	4.2	5.8	4.7	4.5	6.0	7.2
n	9	12	15	12	16	17	11

38. Mean distance from examiner's center to
    subject's center (in millimeters).

If response to item 34 is 2) then complete
items 39-43.

39. A center can be either inferred by the
    point at which the hands are joined or
    by extrapolating the ends of two hands
    which are not joined
    1) yes, a center can be inferred from
       the point of joining of the hands
    2) yes, a center can be extrapolated
       from the ends of two hands that are
       not joined

40. Mean distance of inferred/extrapolated
    center from vertical axis(in millimeters).
    The measurement is assigned a positive value
    if right of the axis or a negative value if
    left of the axis.

41. Mean distance of inferred/extrapolated
    center from the horizontal axis (in
    millimeters). The measurement is assigned
    a positive value if above the axis or a
    negative value if below the axis.

42. Inferred/extrapolated center is in

	20-29	30-39	40-49	50-59	60-69	70-79	80-90
1) upper right	11.1	16.7	40.0	33.3	56.2	17.6	45.5
2) upper left	33.3	16.7	6.7	16.7	18.8	29.4	27.3
3) lower right	22.2	25.0	13.3	25.0		17.6	
4) lower left	22.2	16.7	20.0	8.3		5.9	9.1
5) right axis		8.3		8.3		11.8	
6) left axis	11.1	8.3		8.3			9.1
7) top axis			13.3		12.5		
8) bottom axis		8.3	6.7		12.5	5.9	9.1
9) center						11.8	
n	9	12	15	12	16	17	11

43. Mean distance from examiner's center to inferred/extrapolated center (in millimeters).

	20-29	30-39	40-49	50-59	60-69	70-79	80-90
$\bar{X}$	5.8	4.2	5.2	4.3	5.2	4.7	7.4
SD	4.0	3.1	4.3	2.9	3.8	4.8	6.2
n	9	12	15	12	16	17	11

8:20-EXAMINER CLOCK
Percentage of the Total Number of Subjects Who Made a Given Response

Items 1-17 do not apply to examiner clocks

Hands

Definition of a hand: A line, with or without an arrow, directed toward a number.

		Age Group						
		20-29	30-39	40-49	50-59	60-69	70-79	80-90
18. Two hands present								
1) yes, initially	1	97.5	87.5	90.0	86.5	90.8	79.7	75.6
2) yes, after self-modification	2	2.5	10.0	10.0	11.5	6.6	6.8	9.8
3) no, 2 hands are not present	3							
4) no, 2 hands are not present even after self-modification	4						8.5	12.2
5) 2 hands are present but the time is incorrect	5		2.5		1.9	1.3	3.4	
6) yes, but they are emanating from the 12 position of the clock	6					1.3	1.7	2.4
	n	40	40	40	52	76	59	41

If response in item 18 is 1), 2) or 6) then omit items 19 and 20.

		20-29	30-39	40-49	50-59	60-69	70-79	80-90
19. Hour target number indicated by								
1) minute number written next to hour number (eg. a 10 written adjacent to the 11)	1							40.0
2) a hand	2		100.0		100.0	100.0	28.6	20.0
3) otherwise marked	3						42.9	20.0
4) joined to the minute target number by one line	4						14.3	
5) hour target number not indicated	5							
	2,3							
	1,3							
	n		1		1	1	7	5
20. Minute target number indicated by								
1) a hand	1						14.3	20.0
2) otherwise marked	2						14.3	
3) joined to the hour target number by one line	3							
4) minute target number not indicated	4		100.0		100.0	100.0	71.4	80.0
	n		1		1	1	7	5

21. Proportion of hands

	20-29	30-39	40-49	50-59	60-69	70-79	80-90
1) hour hand longer	7.5	10.0	10.0	9.6	17.1	20.3	19.5
2) minute hand longer	92.5	90.0	90.0	88.5	78.9	69.5	68.3
3) both hands the same length				1.9	3.9	1.7	
4) only one hand present						3.4	4.9
5) not applicable						5.1	7.3
n	40	40	40	52	76	59	41

For items 22 and 23 assign a negative value if the hand is displaced counterclockwise from the target number or a positive value if the hand is displaced clockwise from the target number.

22. Displacement of hour hand/mark from target number in degrees

	20-29	30-39	40-49	50-59	60-69	70-79	80-90
≥-15				1.9			
-12							
-9	5.0	2.5	2.5	1.9	1.3	1.7	
-6	10.0	7.5	20.0	5.8	5.3	3.4	4.9
-3	37.5	20.0	22.5	38.5	43.4	37.3	26.8
0	15.0	22.5	7.5	19.2	2.6	5.1	12.2
+3	7.5	5.0	7.5	11.5	11.8	17.0	24.4
+6	17.5	10.0	15.0	9.6	14.4	20.3	12.2
+9	7.5	20.0	17.5	11.5	14.4	10.2	14.6
+12		7.5	7.5		6.6	5.1	4.8
+15		5.0					
n	40	40	40	52	76	59	41

23. Displacement of minute hand/mark from target number in degrees

	20-29	30-39	40-49	50-59	60-69	70-79	80-90
≥-30							
-15							
-12							
-9	2.5				1.3		
-6	2.5	5.0	2.5	3.8	2.6	1.8	
-3	12.5	17.5	17.5	17.3	7.9	7.1	5.4
0	70.0	55.0	62.5	67.3	59.2	62.5	56.8
+3	10.0	17.5	10.0	7.7	21.0	16.1	21.6
+6	2.5	2.5	7.5	1.9	5.2	7.1	13.5
+9	2.5	2.5		1.9	1.3	1.8	2.7
+12					1.3	3.6	
+15							
+30							
n	40	40	40	52	76	59	41

Items 24 and 25 are to be completed for the Free Drawn Clock and Pre-drawn circle condition only if one or both of the target numbers are spatially incorrect. Items 24 and 25 do not apply to Examiner Clocks.

26. Arrows on hands
    1) arrow on hour hand
    2) arrow on minute hand
    3) arrows on both hands
    4) arrows on neither hand
    5) not applicable - no hands

If response to item 26 is 4) or 5) then omit items 27 and 28.
N.B. (3 mm = 1/8 inch, 6 mm = 1/4 inch)

27. Arrows are displaced from hands by
    1) no displacement
    2) ≤ 4 mm
    3) > 4 mm and ≤ 6 mm
    4) > 6 mm

28. Arrows on hands pointing in the wrong direction
    1) yes
    2) no

29. Any superfluous markings on the clock
    1) yes
    2) no

If response to item 29 is 2) then omit items 30 and 31.

		20-29	30-39	40-49	50-59	60-69	70-79	80-90
26	1				1.9	3.9	3.4	9.8
	2							2.4
	3	77.5	67.5	77.5	76.9	73.7	54.2	41.5
	4	22.5	32.5	22.5	21.2	22.4	37.3	39.0
	5						5.1	7.3
	n	40	40	40	52	76	59	41
27	1	41.9	55.6	51.6	63.4	67.8	67.6	81.8
	2	58.1	40.7	45.2	34.1	28.8	32.4	18.2
	3		3.7	3.2	2.4	3.4		
	4							
	n	31	27	31	41	59	34	22
28	1			3.2		1.7	5.9	
	2	100.0	100.0	96.8	100.0	98.3	94.1	100.0
	n	31	27	31	41	59	34	22
29	1			5.0			1.7	9.8
	2	100.0	100.0	95.0	100.0	100.0	98.3	90.2
	n	40	40	40	52	76	59	41

		20-29	30-39	40-49	50-59	60-69	70-79	80-90
30.	Superfluous lines							
	1) emanating from 12 position of clock						100.0	33.3
	2) 3 hands present							
	3) other superfluous lines							66.7
	4) spokes of a wheel drawn on part of the clock							
	5) spokes of a wheel drawn on the whole clock							
	n						1	3
31.	Miscellaneous markings							
	1) time is written across clock face							
	2) time is written outside of the circle			50.0				
	3) picture of a human face is drawn on clock							
	4) hands with fingers							
	5) markings such as words			50.0				100.0
	6) other							
	n			2				2
	Joining of Hands							
32.	Both hands joined							
	1) yes	67.5	60.0	55.0	42.3	47.4	46.3	38.9
	2) no, mild (<3 mm apart)	22.5	22.5	30.0	38.5	31.6	38.9	41.7
	3) no, moderate (3 mm - 12 mm apart)	10.0	12.5	12.5	15.4	15.8	5.6	11.1
	4) no, severe (>12 mm apart)					1.3	3.7	
	5) yes, but not at the ends		5.0	2.5	3.8	3.9	5.6	8.3
	n	40	40	40	52	76	54	36

N.B.(3 mm = 1/8 inch, 12 mm = 1/2 inch)

If response to item 32 is 1) or 5) then omit item 33.

		20-29	30-39	40-49	50-59	60-69	70-79	80-90
33.	Hands are not joined							
	1) hour hand only emanates from subject's drawn center	46.2	7.1	29.4	25.0	21.6	19.2	36.8
	2) minute hand only emanates from subject's drawn center	7.7	14.3	5.9	14.3	16.2	23.1	31.6
	3) neither hand emanates from subject's drawn center	38.5	35.7	29.4	39.3	45.9	26.9	31.6
	4) not applicable (subject did not draw a center)	7.7	42.9	35.3	21.4	16.2	30.8	
	n	13	14	17	28	37	26	19

Center - If hands are not joined then extrapolate them to create a center for purposes of measurement.

34. Center is drawn by subject

1) yes
2) no, but a center can be extrapolated/inferred by the point at which the hands are joined or by extrapolating the ends of two hands which are not joined
3) no, the hands are not joined, the distance between the ends of the hands is too great to extrapolate a center, or there are not two hands

	20-29	30-39	40-49	50-59	60-69	70-79	80-90
1	82.5	67.5	72.5	76.9	71.1	64.4	80.5
2	17.5	32.5	25.0	23.1	27.6	23.7	12.2
3			2.5		1.3	11.9	7.3
n	40	40	40	52	76	59	41

If response to item 34 is 2) or 3) then omit items 35-38.

35. Mean distance of subject's center from vertical axis (in millimeters). The measurement is assigned a positive value if right of the axis or a negative value if left of the axis.

	20-29	30-39	40-49	50-59	60-69	70-79	80-90
$\bar{X}$	-1.1	.2	-.4	-.6	.2	.1	-.1
SD	1.3	1.8	1.7	1.3	2.1	2.0	1.6
n	33	27	29	40	54	38	33

36. Distance of subject's center from horizontal axis (in millimeters). The measurement is assigned a positive value if above the axis or a negative value if below the axis.

	20-29	30-39	40-49	50-59	60-69	70-79	80-90
$\bar{X}$	1.6	1.3	.2	.9	1.4	1.2	1.6
SD	2.8	2.0	2.1	2.3	2.5	3.2	2.5
n	33	27	29	40	54	38	33

37. Subject's drawn center is in

1) upper right
2) upper left
3) lower right
4) lower left
5) right axis
6) left axis
7) top axis
8) bottom axis
9) center

	20-29	30-39	40-49	50-59	60-69	70-79	80-90
1	6.1	18.5	10.0	15.0	29.1	26.3	21.2
2	48.5	29.6	23.3	22.5	16.4	21.1	15.2
3	3.0	7.4	20.0	2.5		10.5	3.0
4	15.2	7.4	23.3	10.0	10.9	7.9	3.0
5				2.5	9.1	5.3	6.1
6	9.1	3.7	13.3	17.5	5.5	5.3	9.1
7	6.1	18.5	6.7	15.0	18.2	7.9	21.2
8	3.0	3.7		12.5	3.6	13.2	6.1
9	9.1	11.1	3.3	2.5	7.3	2.6	15.2
n	33	27	29	40	54	38	33

38. Distance from examiner's center to subject's center (in millimeters).

	20-29	30-39	40-49	50-59	60-69	70-79	80-90
$\bar{X}$	2.8	2.5	2.2	2.3	2.8	3.3	2.7
SD	2.3	1.5	1.5	1.6	2.3	2.2	2.0
n	33	27	29	40	54	38	33

If response to item 34 is 2) then complete items 39-43.

39. A center can be either inferred by the point at which the hands are joined or by extrapolating the ends of two hands which are not joined
1) yes, a center can be inferred from the point of joining of the hands
2) yes, a center can be extrapolated from the ends of two hands that are not joined

		20-29	30-39	40-49	50-59	60-69	70-79	80-90
39.	1	87.5	50.0	35.7	46.2	63.6	53.3	85.7
	2	12.5	50.0	64.3	53.8	36.4	46.7	14.3
	n	8	14	14	13	22	15	7

40. Distance of inferred/extrapolated center from vertical axis (in millimeters). The measurement is assigned a positive value if right of the axis or a negative value if left of the axis.

		20-29	30-39	40-49	50-59	60-69	70-79	80-90
40.	X̄	-2.5	-1.0	-.4	-.5	.7	3.1	-.8
	SD	1.8	3.6	3.4	4.2	4.1	5.7	2.4
	n	8	14	14	13	22	15	7

41. Distance of inferred/extrapolated center from the horizontal axis (in millimeters). The measurement is assigned a positive value if above the axis or a negative value if below the axis.

		20-29	30-39	40-49	50-59	60-69	70-79	80-90
41.	X̄	3.1	2.3	2.8	1.0	4.0	6.9	9.3
	SD	2.3	7.3	4.0	2.9	9.6	12.0	13.0
	n	8	14	14	13	22	15	7

42. Inferred/extrapolated center is in
1) upper right
2) upper left
3) lower right
4) lower left
5) right axis
6) left axis
7) top axis
8) bottom axis
9) center

		20-29	30-39	40-49	50-59	60-69	70-79	80-90
42.	1		42.9	35.7	30.8	13.6	60.0	28.6
	2	87.5	28.6	14.3	23.1	22.7	13.3	71.4
	3			7.1	15.4	9.1		
	4		21.4	7.1	15.4	9.1	6.7	
	5					13.6	13.3	
	6					4.5		
	7	12.5		14.3	7.7	22.7		
	8			14.3		4.5		
	9		7.1	7.1	7.7		6.7	
	n	8	14	14	13	22	15	7

43. Distance from examiner's center to inferred/extrapolated center (in millimeters).

		20-29	30-39	40-49	50-59	60-69	70-79	80-90
43.	X̄	4.3	6.7	4.7	4.1	7.0	9.9	9.8
	SD	2.2	5.2	3.5	3.1	8.7	11.7	13.3
	n	8	14	14	13	22	15	7

3:00—EXAMINER CLOCK
Percentage of the Total Number of Subjects Who Made a Given Response

Items 1–17 do not apply to examiner clocks

Hands

Definition of a hand: A line, with or without an arrow, directed toward a number.

		Age Group						
		20-29	30-39	40-49	50-59	60-69	70-79	80-90
18. Two hands present								
1) yes, initially	1	100.0	97.5	100.0	94.2	96.1	83.1	78.0
2) yes, after self-modification	2		2.5		5.8	3.9	8.5	9.8
3) no, 2 hands are not present	3							
4) no, 2 hands are not present even after self-modification	4						8.5	12.2
5) 2 hands are present but the time is incorrect	5							
6) yes, but they are emanating from the 12 position of the clock	6							
	n	40	40	40	52	76	59	41

If response in item 18 is 1), 2) or 6) then omit items 19 and 20.

		20-29	30-39	40-49	50-59	60-69	70-79	80-90
19. Hour target number indicated by								
1) minute number written next to hour number (eg. a 10 written adjacent to the 11)	1						60.0	40.0
2) a hand	2						40.0	40.0
3) otherwise marked	3							
4) joined to the minute target number by one line	4							20.0
5) hour target number not indicated	5							
	2,3							
	1,3							
	n						5	5

		20-29	30-39	40-49	50-59	60-69	70-79	80-90
20. Minute target number indicated by								
1) a hand	1						20.0	20.0
2) otherwise marked	2						40.0	20.0
3) joined to the hour target number by one line	3							
4) minute target number not indicated	4						40.0	60.0
	n						5	5

21. Proportion of hands
1) hour hand longer
2) minute hand longer
3) both hands the same length
4) only one hand present
5) not applicable

	20-29	30-39	40-49	50-59	60-69	70-79	80-90
1	5.0	12.5	10.0	13.5	15.8	28.8	31.7
2	95.0	85.0	87.5	84.6	84.2	62.7	53.7
3		2.5	2.5	1.9			2.4
4						3.4	7.3
5						5.1	4.9
n	40	40	40	52	76	59	41

For items 22 and 23 assign a negative value if
the hand is displaced counterclockwise from
the target number or a positive value if the
hand is displaced clockwise from the target
number.

22. Displacement of hour hand/mark from target number in degrees

	20-29	30-39	40-49	50-59	60-69	70-79	80-90
≥-15		2.5					
-12							
-9							
-6	7.5	2.5					
-3	27.5	15.0	2.5	17.3	10.5	13.6	17.1
0	45.0	62.5	32.5	69.2	71.0	72.9	65.9
+3	17.5	12.5	32.5	13.4	14.5	10.2	14.6
+6	2.5	2.5	32.5		3.9	3.4	2.4
+9		2.5					
+12							
+15							
n	40	40	40	52	76	59	41

23. Displacement of minute hand/mark from target number in degrees

	20-29	30-39	40-49	50-59	60-69	70-79	80-90
≥-30							
-15							
-12							
-9							
-6							
-3	12.5	7.5	17.5	5.8	2.6		
0	67.5	67.5	52.5	65.4	73.7	72.0	76.3
+3	20.0	22.5	17.5	25.0	18.4	17.5	21.1
+6		2.5	12.5	1.9	5.3	10.5	2.6
+9				1.9			
+12							
+15							
+30							
n	40	40	40	52	76	57	38

Items 24 and 25 are to be completed for the Free Drawn Clock and Pre-Drawn circle condition only if one or both of the target numbers are spatially incorrect. Items 24 and 25 do not apply to Examiner clocks.

	20-29	30-39	40-49	50-59	60-69	70-79	80-90
26. Arrows on hands							
1) arrow on hour hand				1.9	1.3	3.4	7.3
2) arrow on minute hand							2.4
3) arrows on both hands	77.5	67.5	77.5	76.9	72.4	55.9	43.9
4) arrows on neither hand	22.5	32.5	22.5	21.2	26.3	35.6	41.5
5) not applicable - no hands						5.1	4.9
n	40	40	40	52	76	59	41

If response to item 26 is 4) or 5) then omit items 27 and 28.
N.B.(3 mm = 1/8 inch, 6 mm = 1/4 inch)

	20-29	30-39	40-49	50-59	60-69	70-79	80-90
27. Arrows are displaced from hands by							
1) no displacement	45.2	70.4	48.4	56.1	53.6	77.1	77.3
2) ≤ 4 mm	48.4	29.6	41.9	43.9	44.6	20.0	22.7
3) > 4 mm and ≤ 6 mm	6.5		9.7		1.8	2.9	
4) > 6 mm							
n	31	27	31	41	56	35	22

	20-29	30-39	40-49	50-59	60-69	70-79	80-90
28. Arrows on hands pointing in the wrong direction							
1) yes				2.4	1.8	5.7	
2) no	100.0	100.0	100.0	97.6	98.2	94.3	100.0
n	31	27	31	41	56	35	22

	20-29	30-39	40-49	50-59	60-69	70-79	80-90
29. Any superfluous markings on the clock							
1) yes	2.5	2.5	5.0		1.3		2.4
2) no	97.5	97.5	95.0	100.0	98.7	100.0	97.6
n	40	40	40	52	76	59	41

If response to item 29 is 2) then omit items 30-31.

	20-29	30-39	40-49	50-59	60-69	70-79	80-90
30. Superfluous lines							
1) emanating from 12 position of clock							
2) 3 hands present							
3) other superfluous lines		100.0					
4) spokes of a wheel drawn on part of the clock							
5) spokes of a wheel drawn on the whole clock							
n		1					

31. Miscellaneous markings

	20-29	30-39	40-49	50-59	60-69	70-79	80-90
1) time is written across clock face							
2) time is written outside of the circle							
3) picture of a human face is drawn on clock			50.0				
4) hands with fingers							
5) markings such as words							
6) other	100.0		50.0		100.0		100.0
n	1		2		1		1

Joining of Hands

32. Both hands joined

	20-29	30-39	40-49	50-59	60-69	70-79	80-90
1) yes	67.5	55.0	45.0	34.6	47.4	48.1	50.0
2) no, mild (<3 mm apart)	17.5	25.0	30.0	48.1	27.6	27.8	22.2
3) no, moderate (3 mm – 12 mm apart)	2.5	12.5	2.5	5.8	14.5	16.7	19.4
4) no, severe (>12 mm apart)					1.3	3.7	2.8
5) yes, but not at the ends	12.5	7.5	22.5	11.5	9.2	3.7	5.6
n	40	40	40	52	76	54	36

N.B. (3 mm = 1/8 inch, 12 mm = 1/2 inch)

If response to item 32 is 1) or 5) then omit item 33.

33. Hands are not joined

	20-29	30-39	40-49	50-59	60-69	70-79	80-90
1) hour hand only emanates from subject's drawn center	12.5	26.7	15.4	17.9	12.1	30.8	25.0
2) minute hand only emanates from subject's drawn center	50.0	26.7	46.2	17.9	21.2	11.5	6.3
3) neither hand emanates from subject's drawn center	12.5	26.7	7.7	35.7	39.4	23.1	50.0
4) not applicable (subject did not draw a center)	25.0	20.0	30.8	28.6	27.3	34.6	18.8
n	8	15	13	28	33	26	16

Center – If hands are not joined then extrapolate them to create a center for purposes of measurement.

34. Center is drawn by subject
    1) yes
    2) no, but a center can be extrapolated/ inferred by the point at which the hands are joined or by extrapolating the ends of two hands which are not joined
    3) no, the hands are not joined, the distance between the ends of the hands is too great to extrapolate a center or there are not two hands

If response to item 34 is 2) or 3) then omit items 35-38.

35. Mean distance of subject's center from vertical axis (in millimeters). The measurement is assigned a positive value if right of the axis or a negative value if left of the axis.

36. Distance of subject's center from horizontal axis (in millimeters). The measurement is assigned a positive value if above the axis or a negative value if below the axis.

37. Subject's drawn center is in
    1) upper right
    2) upper left
    3) lower right
    4) lower left
    5) right axis
    6) left axis
    7) top axis
    8) bottom axis
    9) center

		20-29	30-39	40-49	50-59	60-69	70-79	80-90
34.	1	80.0	67.5	67.5	69.2	60.5	54.2	63.4
	2	20.0	32.5	32.5	30.8	38.2	33.9	29.3
	3					1.3	11.9	7.3
	n	40	40	40	52	76	59	41
35.	X̄	-.3	0	-.1	-.1	.2	.3	.1
	SD	1.7	1.3	1.7	1.9	1.6	2.4	1.8
	n	32	27	27	36	46	32	26
36.	X̄	.7	0	-.1	.7	0	.5	.9
	SD	1.8	2.3	1.8	2.2	1.5	2.2	1.7
	n	32	27	27	36	46	32	26
37.	1	28.1	29.6	18.5	22.2	14.9	21.9	19.2
	2	15.6	14.8	18.5	25.0	10.6	6.2	23.1
	3	3.1	14.8	14.8	5.6	6.2	6.2	15.4
	4	12.5	14.8	25.9	11.1	12.8	12.5	3.8
	5		7.4		8.3	14.9	15.6	3.8
	6	28.1	11.1	3.7	13.9	8.5	12.5	7.7
	7	3.1	3.7	7.4	5.6	4.3	15.6	3.8
	8	3.1	3.7	3.7	2.8	4.3	6.2	
	9	6.2		7.4	5.6	14.9	3.1	23.1
	n	32	27	27	36	46	32	26

	20-29	30-39	40-49	50-59	60-69	70-79	80-90

38. Distance from examiner's center to subject's center (in millimeters).

	20-29	30-39	40-49	50-59	60-69	70-79	80-90
$\bar{X}$	2.2	2.1	2.3	2.5	1.7	2.6	2.0
SD	1.5	1.8	1.2	1.6	1.3	1.7	1.8
n	32	27	27	36	46	32	26

If response to item 34 is 2) then complete items 39-43.

39. A center can be either inferred by the point at which the hands are joined or by extrapolating the ends of two hands which are not joined
   1) yes, a center can be inferred from the point of joining of the hands
   2) yes, a center can be extrapolated from the ends of two hands that are not joined

	20-29	30-39	40-49	50-59	60-69	70-79	80-90
1	80.0	71.4	68.7	44.4	69.0	63.6	53.8
2	20.0	28.6	31.3	55.6	31.0	36.4	46.2
n	10	14	16	18	29	22	13

40. Distance of inferred/extrapolated center from vertical axis (in millimeters). The measurement is assigned a positive value if right of the axis or a negative value if left of the axis.

	20-29	30-39	40-49	50-59	60-69	70-79	80-90
$\bar{X}$	.6	1.9	.1	.6	2.4	1.3	1.3
SD	1.5	2.5	2.0	3.2	3.2	2.6	4.0
n	10	14	16	18	29	22	13

41. Distance of inferred/extrapolated center from the horizontal axis (in millimeters). The measurement is assigned a positive value if above the axis or a negative value if below the axis.

	20-29	30-39	40-49	50-59	60-69	70-79	80-90
$\bar{X}$	-.8	-1.3	-1.5	.4	-.7	-1.8	.5
SD	1.8	3.6	1.6	1.8	2.2	3.0	2.9
n	10	14	16	18	29	22	13

42. Inferred/extrapolated center is in

	20-29	30-39	40-49	50-59	60-69	70-79	80-90
1) upper right	10.0	21.4	12.5	11.1	20.7	9.1	7.7
2) upper left	30.0	28.6	31.3	16.7	3.4	4.5	30.8
3) lower right	10.0	7.1	18.8	11.1	37.9	45.5	30.8
4) lower left		14.3	6.2	22.2	6.9	9.1	7.7
5) right axis				11.1	13.8	9.1	7.7
6) left axis	10.0		6.2	5.6	3.4	4.5	7.7
7) top axis	20.0	7.1		16.7			7.7
8) bottom axis	20.0	14.3	25.0				
9) center		7.1		5.6	13.8	18.2	
n	10	14	16	18	29	22	13

43. Distance from examiner's center to infered/extrapolated center (in millimeters).

	20-29	30-39	40-49	50-59	60-69	70-79	80-90
$\overline{X}$	1.9	4.0	2.6	2.8	3.9	3.6	4.1
SD	1.4	3.0	1.6	2.5	2.8	2.6	3.0
n	10	14	16	18	29	22	13

Index

Page numbers followed by f indicate figures. Page numbers followed by t indicate tables.